The Forager's Cookbook

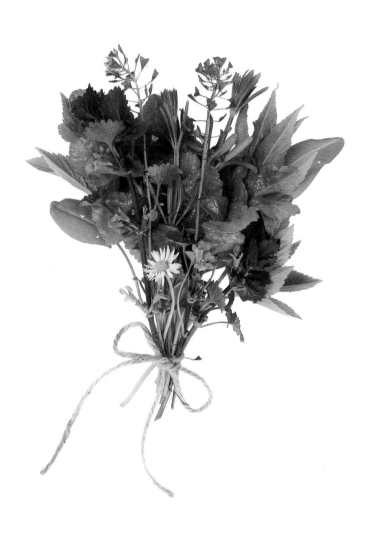

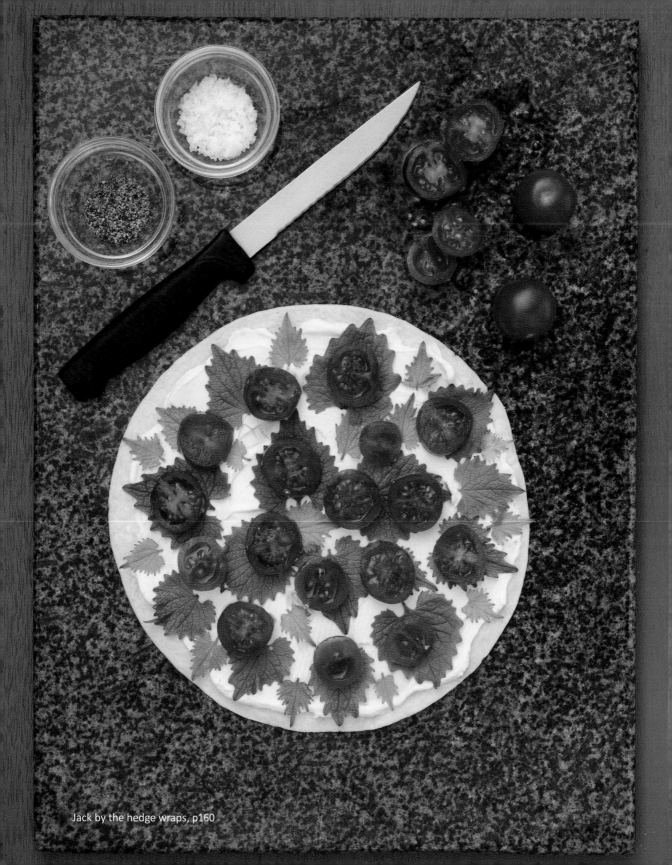

Jack by the hedge wraps, p160

The
Forager's Cookbook
Identify & Prepare Edible Weeds & Wild Plants

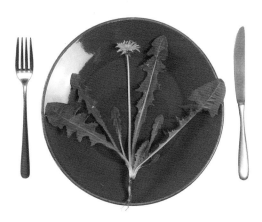

Julie Bruton-Seal & Matthew Seal

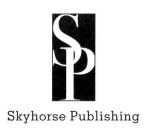

Skyhorse Publishing

Skyhorse Publishing books may be purchased in bulk at special discounts for sales promotion, corporate gifts, fund-raising, or educational purposes. Special editions can also be created to specifications. For details, contact the Special Sales Department, Skyhorse Publishing, 307 West 36th Street, 11th Floor, New York, NY 10018 or info@skyhorsepublishing.com.

Skyhorse® and Skyhorse Publishing® are registered trademarks of Skyhorse Publishing, Inc.®, a Delaware corporation.

Visit our website at www.skyhorsepublishing.com.

10 9 8 7 6 5 4 3 2 1

Library of Congress Cataloging-in-Publication Data is available on file.

Cover design by David Ter-Avanesyan
Cover photographs by Julie Bruton-Seal

Print ISBN: 978-1-5107-7295-3
Ebook ISBN: 978-1-5107-7486-5

Printed in China

Please note:

The herbal information in *The Forager's Cookbook* is compiled from a blend of historical and modern sources, from folklore and personal experience. If you have a medical condition, consult a professional herbalist. Heed the cautions given, and take particular care if you are pregnant. When trying a new food for the first time, experiment with a small amount initially to make sure it doesn't disagree with you, and be certain of your identification before ingesting anything.

Contents

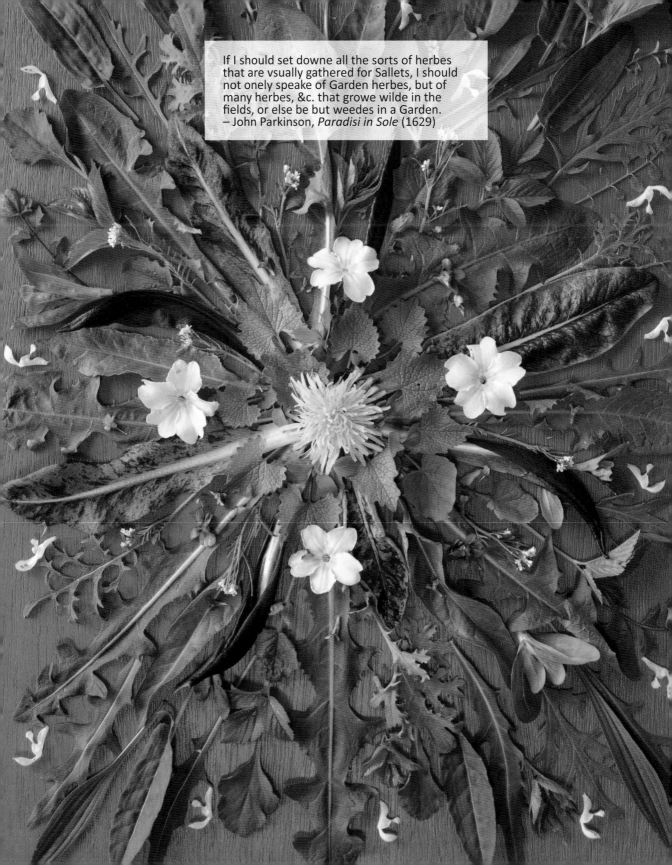

If I should set downe all the sorts of herbes that are vsually gathered for Sallets, I should not onely speake of Garden herbes, but of many herbes, &c. that growe wilde in the fields, or else be but weedes in a Garden.
— John Parkinson, *Paradisi in Sole* (1629)

Preface & Acknowledgments

This book is a celebration of weeds, the resilient wild plants that have learned to live alongside humans and travel the world with them. These are companions of our backyard and probably yours too, though you may not have thought of them before now as sources of delicious food.

The title and full idea for the book arrived in a dream of Julie's in October 2019, and we began work. We have long admired the strengths and virtues of our common weeds, and wanted to get to know them better. After much thought, we chose 23 plants and a mushroom that are common in the temperate world, and which we found tasty to eat in various forms. We also wanted to offer in-depth plant biographies to accompany the recipes, giving some idea of how certain weeds have been so successful.

Weeds are hated by gardeners, especially ground elder and honey mushroom, and in practice are almost impossible to get rid of. If you are stuck with these tenacious life forms, perhaps it's time to appreciate their good side – if you can't beat them, eat them!

Weeds are defined as plants in the wrong place, as outcasts, not welcome in our fields and gardens. But consider, there is no botanical family called weeds; a weed is a purely human construct. They are subject to our 'plant blindness', being too much under our noses to have been thought useful at all, while we look to exotic plants from far away. If we notice weeds at all, it is as enemies – they are in our way, whether farmer or gardener, and we are out to destroy them, always destroy.

It's a mindset that we think needs to change. We propose that weeds can be a useful free food resource, a garden microcrop. They can and should be a delicious, local and sustainable addition to our everyday cuisine, offering us exciting new flavors. They are there as survival food if we need it, and grow happily without any help from us.

Like every project this one has deeper roots too. Julie has been co-author of a plant-based recipe book before, working with her friend Carol Tracy in the 1980s on *Vegetarian Masterpieces*. Self-published in spiral-bound format in Charlotte NC, it went into at least ten printings.

Matthew has another route into the present book. He remembers his father, George Seal, buying Sir Edward Salisbury's *Weeds & Aliens* book in the New Naturalist series, when it appeared in 1961, for the then hefty price of 30 shillings (closer to $35 today).

The book itself revealed somebody taking weeds seriously and doing amazing research on plants that were usually dismissed, not discussed. Somewhere along the line Matthew 'acquired' the book, and it has been a background resource in the present project.

All of our previous five books together have featured recipes, whether 'receipts' in the old sense of herbal preparations or the modern notion of instructions for cooking food. The present book is really an extension of our recipe-making rather than a departure, with the subject matter now domestic weeds and the food recipes specifically plant-based.

Recipes can seldom be wholly original but we have taken inspiration from cuisines worldwide, and have tried to give a wide variety of ways to enjoy our chosen weeds. We hope readers will be inspired to embark on careful culinary experiments with their own local weed flora.

We have tested all the recipes for ourselves, the process of collecting, cooking and photographing them testing – and rewarding – our patience and hunger pangs.

We have had enthusiastic support from friends, family and colleagues in tasting our food or our words. We particularly thank Jen Bartlett, Andrew Chevallier, Kaz da Silva, Maria Davidson, Charlotte du Cann, Mark Fairhead, Christina Gathergood, Fred Gillam, Christine Herbert, Valerie Macfarlane, Anne Roy, Helen Seal, Ruby Taylor and Monica Wilde. Needless to say, we alone take full responsibility for the contents.

All the photographs are by Julie, except for the author photo taken by Tarl Bruton. We thank the John Innes Foundation Collection of Rare Botanical Books, Norwich, for permission to reproduce the image of plantain by Maria Merian (1717).

Julie Bruton-Seal & Matthew Seal
Ashwellthorpe, Norfolk, January 2022

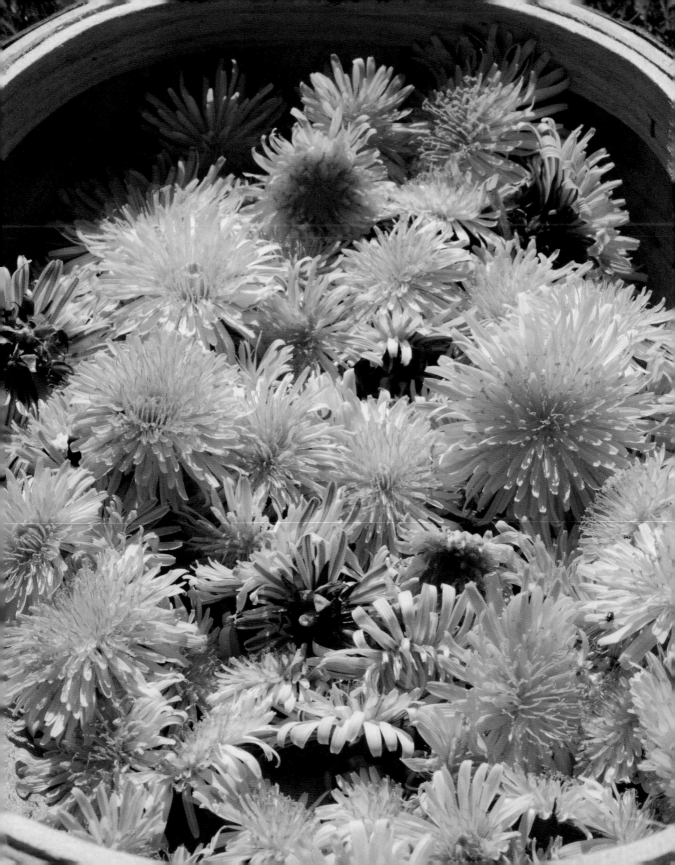

Introduction

Why should we eat our weeds? Because they are delicious, adding a palate of new flavors in everyday cooking. They are also nutritious and too good to waste.

Weeds are actually more nutritious than most of the vegetables we grow or buy. They often have deep roots that loosen the soil and bring minerals up from far below. Weeds can help cover the soil, keep moisture in it and preserve its fertility.

They offer a second crop among our other plants, for free, and are often available in the late winter and early spring when our vegetables are yet to get going. When it's time to weed, the edible weeds can be eaten. Why throw perfectly good food on the compost heap?

Weeds are strong and resilient, and can survive the vagaries of climate change better than our pampered crops. We now know that a greater diversity of plants enhances life in the soil, which in turn makes the soil more fertile and more able to hold water and to sequester greenhouse gases. Healthier soil means healthier food and healthier people.

Plants have been growing on Earth for millions of years, while we as humans are very recent arrivals. Weeds are the plants that have best adapted to our presence and activities, particularly since we adopted agriculture about 10,000 years ago. They have been our constant companions, but our relationship with them has usually been toxic and destructive.

Weeds are amazing beings that we have failed to see.

Weeds and weedness

Please don't dismiss weeds as weedy. 'Weedy' or 'weediness' imply something weak, spindly, rather useless. In fact weeds are exactly the opposite.

People used to think that cleavers, for example, was weak because it draped itself over other vegetation. Scientists now say its stems have the highest breaking strains yet recorded in a land-based plant, and it has complex differential upper and lower spinal arrays, allowing it to cling or release as needed.

Since 'weediness' is no longer a useful term we propose using **weedness** to describe the many features of weeds that make them so capable of survival. For instance, we identify seventeen measures of weedness for blackberry, king of weeds in our garden.

We invite you to see weeds in another light, to see them at all in fact.

We moderns do suffer plant blindness, and it's a matter of re-education – weeducation, we'd say, tongue in cheek – to recover a form of seeing that we have lost. Gardeners are more likely than the general population to notice plants, but many weeds only make them 'see red' and think murderous thoughts.

We appreciate it is a big 'ask' to look at weeds as having any positive value, let alone eat them, but we think the effort will repay you. Others have made the same journey.

'I will stop to notice thee'

The English poet John Clare (1793–1864) had deep weed (in)sight. He was a farm laborer, a 'weeder' in his own words, and he loved 'all wild flowers (none are weeds with me)' – for biography, see Bate 2004.

Clare's poem 'To an Insignificant Flower, obscurely blooming in a lonely wild' (1820) begins

> And though thou seem'st a weedling wild,
> Wild and neglected like me,
> Thou still art dear to Nature's child,
> And I will stop to notice thee.

First is stopping and noticing 'an insignificant flower'. Then comes the belief that a humble weed can be the match of any garden flower:

> For oft, like thee, in wild retreat,
> Array'd in humble garb like thee,
> There's many a seeming weed proves sweet,
> As sweet as garden-flowers can be.

Then empathy can grow. Without 'improvement' (cultivation), the 'seeming' weed is 'wild and neglected like me', he writes:

> And, like to thee, each seeming weed
> Flowers unregarded; like to thee,
> Without improvement, runs to seed,
> Wild and neglected like me.

Clare could just about hold together (at least in the first part of his life) his daily toil of hoeing weeds while taking time to name, versify and appreciate them.

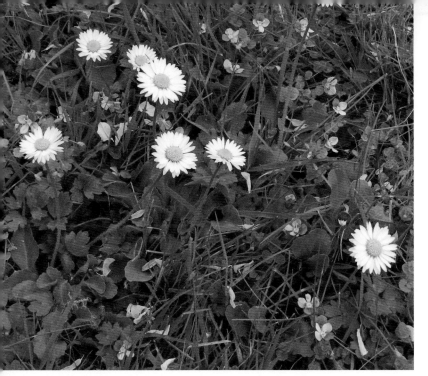

Daisies and speedwell
flowering in a spring lawn

*The same wild integrity that
exists in plants growing in
pristine wilderness areas is
also found in the nature of
the wild weeds growing in
open lands around and in
the margins of civilization.
Wild weeds have an intrinsic
wisdom for resilience and
have mastered their abilities
of survival.*
– Blair (2014)

*Mowing the grass once a
fortnight in pleasure grounds,
as now practiced, is a costly
mistake. We want shaven
carpets of grass here and
there, but what nonsense it is
to shave it as often as foolish
men shave their faces! ...
Who would not rather see the
waving grass with countless
flowers than a close surface
without a blossom?*
– Robinson (1895)

Identify & destroy?

What of us two centuries on? Ever since humans began manipulating the environment for our own ends, we have been editing out the plants that aren't useful to us. Over time we came to see weeds as competition for the plants we wanted to grow. We now know that plant relationships are far more complex than that, with soil life, particularly fungal networks, connecting everything in an entangled web of interactions.

In modern-day chemicalized agriculture, weeds in mono-crops are often exterminated with herbicides. Gardeners also use chemicals to keep things tidy. The problem is that glyphosate (Roundup®), one of the most widely used weed killers, wipes out soil micro-organisms and damages our own vital microbiome.

We aren't saying weeds should be left to take over the world, but believe that a better balance can be reached. If you are a gardener with an abundance of ground elder, you are never likely to be able to eradicate it, so why not live with it and learn to appreciate it by using it for food, medicine and flower arrangements?

We believe a lawn full of dandelions, daisies, plantain, yarrow and other plants is far more useful and interesting than a mown green grass monoculture.

Within the balance you draw for yourself we hope you can find a space to recognize your weeds and have an ongoing relationship that includes eating them and ingesting their powerful zest for life. Indeed, all green plants are embodied light.

Weeds are free, local and sustainable, and they grow, an unused, unseen resource, without us needing to do a thing.

Identify & harvest

With weeds, as with all wild plants you may be planning to eat, proper ID is essential. Rule number one is eat only what you are sure of.

We have provided clear photographs and other written identification details for all the weeds in this book. If you are unfamiliar with these plants you may also wish to have a field guide.

In the UK, try, for example, the photographic floras of Simon Harrap (2013) or Roger Phillips (1986), or the floral paintings of Marjorie Blamey (2003) – see References at the back of the book – or many another. Wherever you live you can find local equivalents.

Best of all, locate a teacher who can introduce you to any unfamiliar plants. Take any opportunity you can to go on herb walks. Contact an herbalist or forager local to you, by word of mouth or with a local foraging organization. If you take your children on plant walks you could be giving them a gift for life.

If you see a plant often enough, and get close to it, touching and smelling, and best of all drawing it and sitting with it, you begin to know the way it carries itself, its form. In other words, you learn and intuit what the birders call 'jizz'. Once knowing your plant's jizz you can even recognize it from the car as it flashes by out the window (be careful, though, such botanizing could become a dangerous habit!).

Remember that when digging up a plant, including a weed, if it is not on your land you need permission. In practice people might be happy for you to collect their weeds – they might even pay you to weed for them!

We give guidance on gathering/ harvesting in each chapter but heed the general point to avoid plants that might have been treated with pesticides or other chemicals, or those close by the road. Of course, if picking weeds from your own garden, as we have done, you will already know whether they are organic and clean.

Weedness & bitterness

As part of becoming co-workers with your weeds we thought it useful to offer you extensive biographies of the weed subjects we have chosen. A plant like nipplewort, say, makes for wonderful eating but is relatively little known or appreciated.

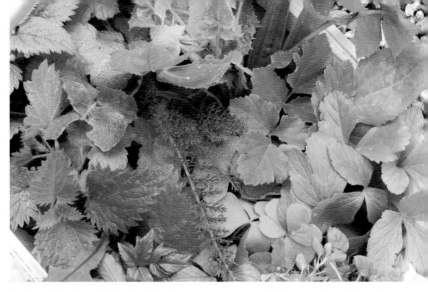

Winter weeds: gathered abundance in our garden on a mild day in January

So in each of our 22 main chapters we begin with a section on weedness ('what kind of a weed is …?'), followed by other sections related to history, uses, and gathering and cooking.

The weeds we have selected are the ones that grow around us, and that we like to eat. There are many more edible weeds, but most of the plants we have featured are worldwide weeds, found extensively in temperate regions.

Weeds, like other wild plants, will often have stronger flavors than we are used to. Most modern vegetables have been

There is a sort of sacredness about them [weeds]. Perhaps if we could penetrate Nature's secrets we should find that what we call weeds are more essential to the well-being of the world than the most precious fruit or grain.
– Hawthorne (1869)

It would appear that at the moment many plants are beginning to speak up for themselves and call our attention to the fact that we have been completely ignoring them as weeds, or as rather insignificant local, outdated beings that have been superseded by the exotic exciting new favorites, often from overseas, often packaged as products.
– Darrell (2020)

Rebel botanical chalkers

France has taken a lead in banning herbicide and pesticide uses in public places (2017), and extended the ban to private gardens (2019). An unexpected outcome of these initiatives is a rising number of 'rebel botanists' internationally who delight in chalking the common names of weeds and pavement plants right alongside them. They then share the images on social media.

Hooray! A new visibility for the downtrodden and ignored flora of our streets. In London a French botanist, Sophie Leguil, has set up a More Than Weeds campaign and has secured the council's permission to chalk the names of wild plants on the pavements of Hackney.

Usually this is illegal. Chalking on the pavement for hopscotch or naming weeds can land you with a fine of up to £2,500. Just let them try, we say! Meanwhile, as Leguil points out, 'We talk a lot about plant blindness – what if putting names on plants could make people look at them in a different way? … I despair at how sanitized London has become.'

Source: Alex Morss, *Guardian*, 1 May 2020; updates in morethanweeds.co.uk, Le plan Ecophto II+, ecologie.gouv.fr.

[there remains] a creeping garden beneath us, seeking an opportunity to flourish in the cracks of things we build.
– Rees (2019)

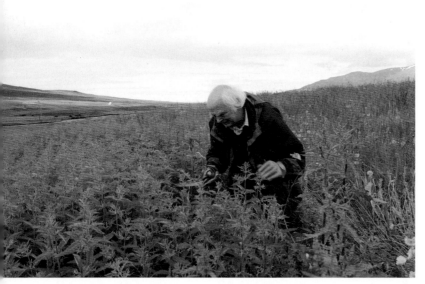

Matthew practicing what he preaches: rather gingerly picking nettles in Iceland

The most important flowers in the world are not those Wordsworth saw – that sea of golden daffodils. It's the one dandelion at the bus stop, the one brave soul poking out of the concrete. It's the pure, simple beauty of nature, like the blackbird's song.
– Packham (2021)

As you learn and forage new plants it is important (and fun) to take the time to experiment with them. … Plantain can be turned into 'seaweed' … stinging nettles are beautiful and crunchy once fried and sprinkled with wild spices … curly dock leaves can become sushi wraps. … I tell my students that they don't have to think outside of the box but can simply eliminate the box altogether! Think freely! Many edible foraged plants have culinary uses that are begging to be discovered.
– Baudar (2016)

bred to taste more bland than their wild ancestors. This is particularly true of bitter flavors. Bitterness is a virtue in our book(s), as it was in ancient Japan, where *sansai* was the term used for 'mountain vegetables' or foraged wild plants.

Bitterness as a taste is linked to good liver health, and bitter flavors stimulate digestion. Persist, and your taste buds will soon adapt and learn to welcome any extra bitterness that your weed meals give you.

We actually know very little of the chemistry of the plants we eat. Yes, there is data about the proteins, carbohydrates, fats and a few vitamins and minerals, and we generally have some idea of the calories certain foods provide. But plants and fungi (and their bacterial companions) produce a vast array of other compounds that contribute to their nutritional value and are vital for good health.

Overall, weeds and wild foods are nutritionally dense, which means you will need to eat less of them to feel sated. Stick with these wild tastes because you are taking in the plant's wildness, its survival strength.

Be aware that weeds can vary in their flavors from one place or terroir to another, and at different times of year. Experiment with this diversity.

A note on presentation

We have our own style of presenting recipes, integrating ingredients and instructions into running sentences. We highlight ingredients in **bold** type. We feel this method is closer to how cooking actually takes place. A few cookbooks adopt this same style, and we find it much easier than having to go back and forth between a list of ingredients and the instructions.

We have taken inspiration from around the world for our plant-based recipes, and have tried to include a wide variety, both savory and sweet, for food and drink, snacks or main meals.

Our recipes are generally quite simple, but they can be adapted and amended to suit your own preferences. Many can be used with other edible weeds than the ones we have chosen, and we encourage you to improvize once you learn to identify them confidently.

Get to know each plant through the seasons, and use your imagination to concoct your own recipes.

The old definition of weeds is that they are plants growing in the wrong place, from a human point of view. We are saying they are actually in just the right place, in our garden, for us to harvest.

We hope this book will inspire you to look at weeds with new eyes, as free ingredients for a venture into culinary ecology, as well as appreciate them for their own sake.

Measurements

We have given both metric and US cup measurements. The cups are standard measuring cups, with dry ingredients being measured level. The exact size of your measuring cup (US or UK) doesn't matter as long as you use it consistently – it is the proportions that matter.

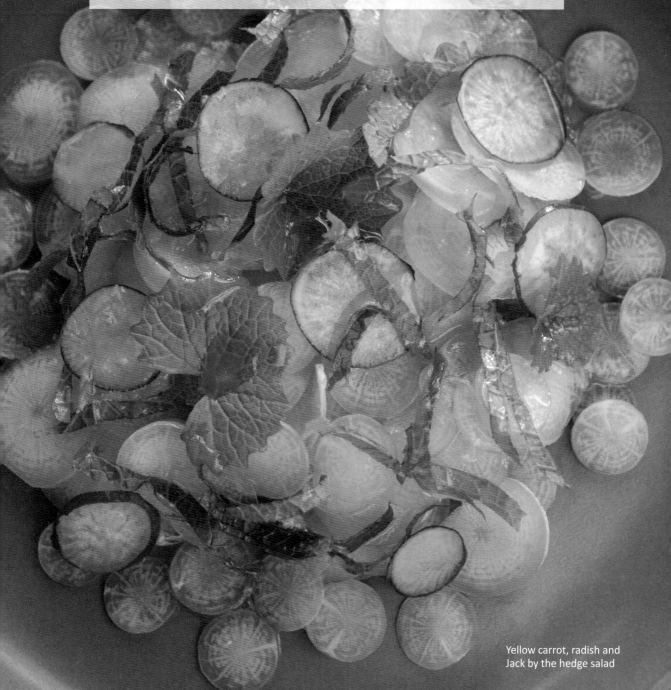

The
Forager's Cookbook

Yellow carrot, radish and
Jack by the hedge salad

Alexanders

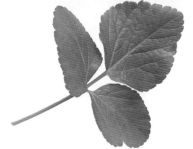

Alexanders (*Smyrnium olusatrum*) is a tall biennial (two-year lifespan) member of the Apiaceae (carrot family). Historically, it spread from the Mediterranean and made the switch from wild-gathered plant to garden crop, and back to wild. It was both food and medicine in Classical and medieval times. Losing out to celery as a salad crop from the 16th century, it is making a comeback as a winter-foraged wild food. The best eating is when leaves and buds are young and tender; the inner stem and roots can be braised or sautéed.

**Apiaceae
(Umbelliferae)
Carrot family**

Biennial. Dies back completely in summer, and reappears in autumn with lush light green growth.

Edible parts: Young leaves in winter; buds, flowers, stems and roots in spring; seeds in late summer.

Distinguishing features: Alexanders has smooth <u>shiny</u> three-lobed leaves; <u>smooth</u>, hairless and hollow flower stalk; grows to over 1m (3.3ft), with umbels of small <u>yellow flowers</u> appearing in spring, followed by large seeds, which ripen to black.

In the eastern half of North America the related golden alexanders (*Zizea aurea*) is an abundant native plant of woodlands. Named for German botanist Johann Baptist Ziz and *aurea* (golden), it is a perennial and smaller than alexanders, with more slender flowers and less blowsy leaves that go purple. Golden alexanders is edible in the same way as alexanders, but some foragers urge caution in eating its roots.

Caution: Avoid large quantities during pregnancy

What kind of a weed is alexanders?

Geoffrey Grigson, writing in 1955, says alexanders is *happiest and most frequent by the sea*. He's right, and sturdy stands of this vigorous and stately umbellifer proliferate in sheltered cliff and roadsides near eastern and southern coasts of Britain and Ireland, often on small islands. It is a scarce coastal species in parts of North America.

It also seems to be pressing inland, at least in our part of East Anglia, thriving in hedgerows some 55km (35 miles) from the Norfolk coast, and in gardens. The picture opposite shows alexanders by our garden shed. We sowed a few seeds in our garden some years ago, and it's now a winter weed with us.

Look at the rootstock, spreading as wide as a fist with a taproot several feet deep (see p17), and the chest-high mass of stems and broad leaves, and you see why it can crowd out even its cousin hogweed. Alexanders is a biennial, and the first year of its life is spent building up that stealthy root system; the second year is given over to flowering, setting seed and then dying.

Our region is more or less at the northern edge of its wild-growing range. If it is spreading inland at a measurable rate it is also moving ever earlier in its growing habits. In a 17th-century herbal like that of John Parkinson (1640), alexanders is said to flower in June and July; we often have plants blooming in March.

It is an early responder to climate change, giving it competitive advantages over other plants and a nudge to us. In winter and early spring there isn't a wealth of plants to gather, and foragers are taking the culinary hint. Alexanders is robust and can fill the 'hunger gap'.

The history of alexanders

The scientific and common names are clearly Mediterranean. Archaeological finds suggest it was cultivated in Iron Age Greece (c1300–700BC), and the earliest written reference is in Theophrastus, the Greek 'father of botany' (c371–c287BC).

Its roots and shoots had become a popular potherb and vegetable by the time of Alexander the Great in the 4th century BC. The English name Alexanders could be for the emperor, or indeed for the port in Egypt that he founded and which bore his name.

The plant's Greek name *hipposelinon* means 'horse parsley or celery', while Columella, the Roman agricultural writer (AD4–70), knew alexanders as 'myrrh of Achaea', the then Latin

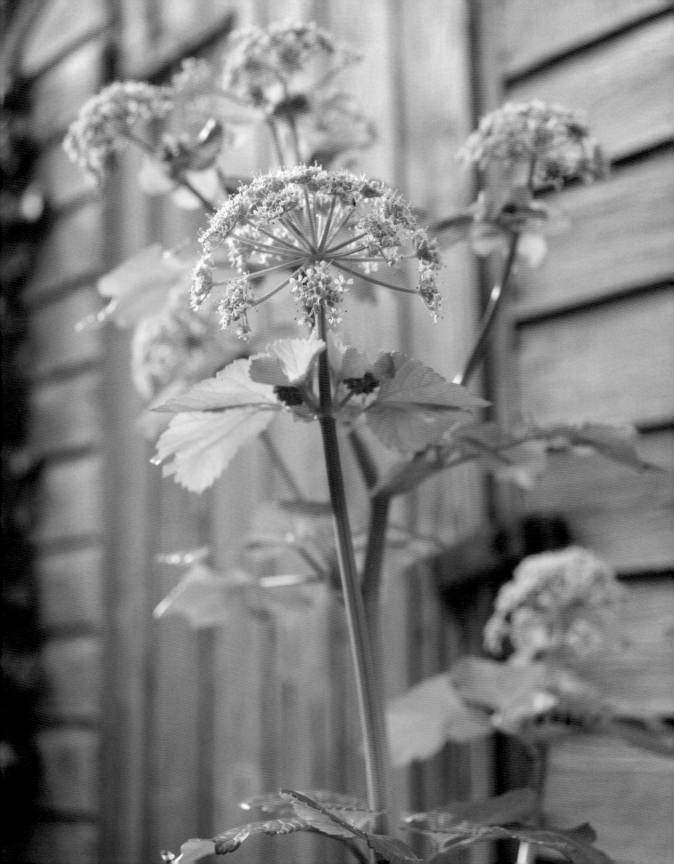

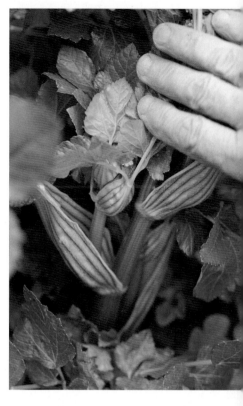

Ripe seeds of alexanders; right: flower buds, showing the characteristic striped leaf bases that enclose them until they emerge

Its certain aromatic or pungent flavor ... would be too strong for modern tastes.
– Pratt (1866)

... a timely potherb.
– Lawson (1618)

[broth of alexanders] ... *which although it be a little bitter, yet it is both wholsome, and pleasing to a great many, by reason of the aromaticall or spicie taste, warming and comforting the stomack, and helping it digest the many waterish and flegmaticke meates* [that] *are in those times* [spring] *much eaten.*
– Parkinson (1629)

name for Greece. A contemporary of Columella, the natural history writer Pliny (AD23/24–79), called it *olusatrum*, or 'black (pot)herb', the species name Linnaeus would choose for it in the mid-18th century. Pliny thought it *a herb of exceptionally remarkable nature*, and noted another name, *zmyrnium*, a reference to myrrh, the reputed taste of the plant's juice.

The myrrh reference has followed the plant in its modern generic form *Smyrnium*. Some people do find the taste and scent myrrh-like, especially of the flower stalk, though others get more lovage in it; an old common name is black lovage.

There are as yet no British archaeological records of alexanders before the Roman invasion in AD43, but in 1911 seeds were found in a Roman-era well near Chepstow.

The consensus is that alexanders was among the plants that accompanied the Roman imperial takeover of Western Europe and North Africa. Some say the Romans used it as fodder for their horses as well as a boiled vegetable, a broth or the seeds as a condiment.

As both food and medicine alexanders continued to be a widely grown monastic plant in medieval times. Many scattered inland sightings of it in Britain relate to sites of kitchen gardens of former monastic houses.

By the time of the dissolution of the monasteries in the 1530s and 1540s, wild celery (*Apium graveolens*) was starting to be transformed by Italian agronomists into the blanched cultivated salad plant we know today.

Around Europe celery's milder taste came to be favored over the stronger charms of alexanders, which lost popularity. In our own times alexanders is being newly appraised as a forageable weed.

Herbal & other uses of alexanders

Alexanders was classified as 'hot and dry in the third degree', and its actions were accordingly forceful. It was found to work strongly on the urinary and digestive systems, especially the seeds.

The English writer William Salmon (1710) summed up: *alexanders effectually provokes Urine, helps the Strangury, and prevails against Gravel and Tartarous Matter in Reins and Bladder.* In modern terms, he was calling it a diuretic, which cleared the urinary system, including kidney and bladder stones.

Roman writers knew alexanders as an emmenagogue, a herb to promote menstruation. Salmon confirmed that the plant *powerfully provokes the Terms*; it also *expels the Birth* (afterbirth). That is, it was and is a powerful uterine tonic, and should still be treated with caution during pregnancy.

Medieval root broths, made up of alexanders, celery, fennel and parsley, were used as purgatives for sluggish stomachs in the spring.

Alexanders was an 'official' herb of the apothecaries in the first London *Pharmacopoeia* (1618). But by Salmon's herbal nearly a century later it had gone; he noted *The Shops* [ie apothecaries] *keep nothing of this plant.*

It was sliding out of favor in both medicine and cooking, though there are records of alexanders root sold for urinary problems in Covent Garden market in the late 18th century.

Of course, it does not follow that because alexanders has gone out of fashion it is no longer useful as a backyard medicine. The virtues the old herbalists championed remain valid, and clinical experimentation is opening up some intriguing new possibilities.

One is alexanders' essential oil. Italian researchers in 2014 found that oil from the flowers induces apoptosis, or cell death, in human colon carcinoma cells. A 2017 finding is that this oil may be effective against the protozoal parasite causing African trypanosomiasis.

How to eat alexanders

Alexanders is also there to be eaten! It has a strong taste for our bland modern palates, which will usually prefer celery and parsnip to alexanders and lovage.

We find alexander leaves have a strong celery taste, and, like celery, quickly become stringy, so are best used young and in moderation. We use the taste to good effect to flavor salt (see p20).

Once the plant produces flower buds, the flavor of these and the stems is much milder and more floral. Larger stems need peeling. The flower buds and young stalks are tasty cooked with broccoli. They can also be used in sweet dishes and combine well with rhubarb or angelica.

The roots can be cooked like parsnips but usually have a stronger taste.

The simplest recipe of all is to collect the black seeds, and dry and grind them, either manually in a pepper mill or electrically in a coffee mill. Treat the seeds as a black pepper-like condiment and invite them onto your table; the urban forager John Rensten (2016) uses the seeds to replace pepper in his wild chai recipe.

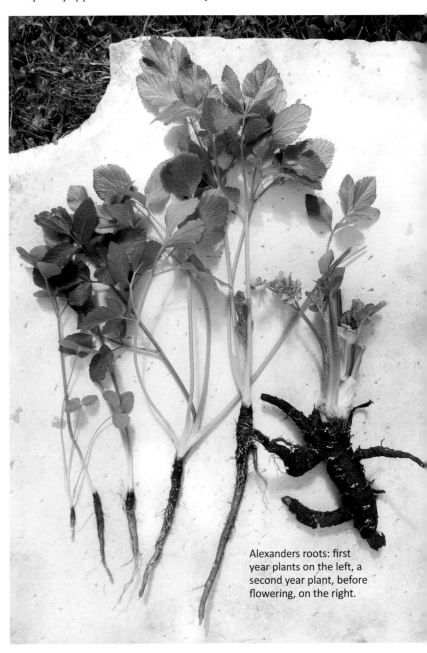

Alexanders roots: first year plants on the left, a second year plant, before flowering, on the right.

Alexanders **Tempura**

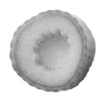

Alexanders makes great tempura. You can use the leaf stalks during autumn and winter before they get too fibrous, soaking them to make them curl beautifully, or use the peeled flower stems cut into rings in spring. Both are delicious, but with subtle differences in flavor.

For the **alexanders leaf stalks**, cut them into roughly 8cm (3in) lengths and cut two or three slits about a centimeter (½in) into each end. Discard any that seem too stringy. Leave in **cold water** overnight or until the ends have curled as much as you want them to.

Pick the **alexanders flower stalks** while the plant is in bud, before the flowers open. Peel to remove the stringy bits and cut them into rings.

For the tempura batter, mix equal parts **flour** and **cornstarch** and mix with **cold water** to the thickness of cream, just thick enough to thinly coat the alexanders when they are dipped into it.

Roll the alexanders in **flour**, then dip into the batter. Shake off excess batter, and deep fry in **vegetable oil** until golden.

Variations: You can use use sparkling water instead of plain water in the tempura batter.

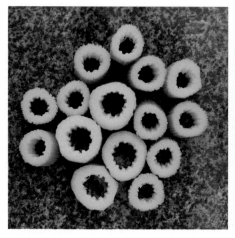

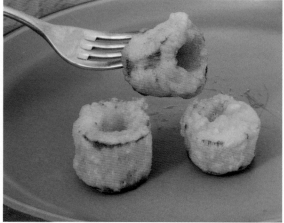

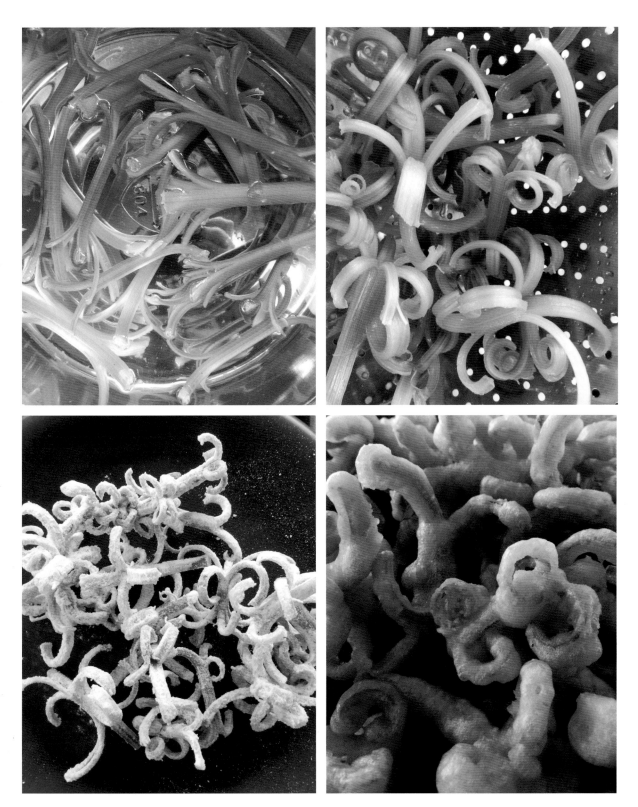

Alexanders Salt

This method can be used for many of the weeds in this book. We've used it most often with alexanders, nettle and ground elder.

The initial step is to dry your herb, then powder it – a clean coffee grinder works well. The powder can be sieved to remove any larger bits that didn't get powdered. The herb powders can be used as they are, to add to recipes or sprinkle on food, or made into this flavored salt.

Mix **1 part ground dried alexanders tops**
with **4 parts coarse salt (we used grey French sea salt)**
and **1 part water**, adding just enough to moisten the other ingredients.

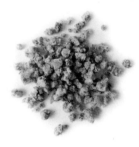

Leave to sit for half an hour or so, then spread out on a tray in a dehydrator or a cool oven to dry, crumbling it with your fingers from time to time as it dries so that you don't get big clumps of salt.

Store in an airtight jar.

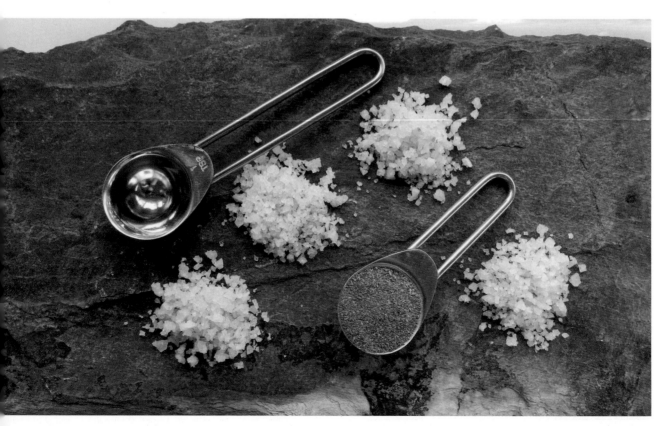

Alexanders & Red Cabbage **Slaw**

This is a wonderful winter salad. Alexanders comes into its own when there isn't much fresh greenery to be found. We usually blanch the alexanders to tone down the taste a little, but if your leaves are very young and tender and you like the flavor, use them raw.

For 4 to 6 people.

Blanch **a few handfuls of alexanders leaves** in **boiling water** for about a minute. Older leaves may need a little longer. Taste to check. Drain and drop immediately into **cold water**.

Mix together in a bowl: **1 cup chopped blanched alexanders, 4 cups finely mandolined red cabbage** and **1 finely sliced apple**, cut into slivers.

Toss with about 4 tablespoons of dressing – use your favorite, or our recipe below.

Top with **a handful of toasted pumpkin seeds**, and serve with more on the side.

Dressing (put in a jam jar and shake):
**188ml (¾ cup) rapeseed oil
60ml (¼ cup) white wine vinegar
1 tablespoon orange zest
3 tablespoons orange juice
1 tablespoon lemon juice**

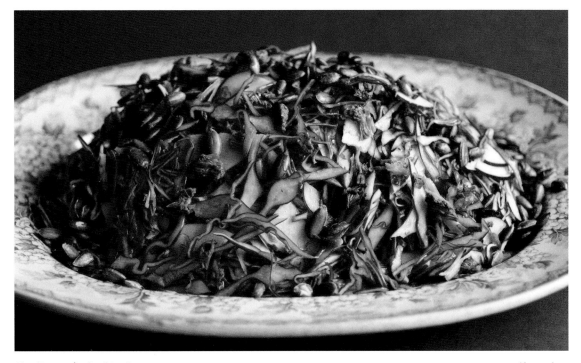

Alexanders Stems

Alexanders flower stems are best harvested just before the flowers open. They need to be peeled, and are then very tender and succulent. The flavor is less like celery than the leaves and more fragrant, like angelica.

They can be used in either sweet or savory dishes, including the tempura on p18. Try simply braising them with a little garlic and oil. They make a tasty syrup with sugar and lemon juice.

The stems combine very well with rhubarb. Peel the **alexanders stems** and remove any stringy bits from the **rhubarb**. Cut into chunks and place in a baking dish.

Sprinkle with **brown sugar or coconut blossom sugar**, cover with a lid or foil, and bake at 175C/350F for about an hour or until they are tender. They are delicious as is, or add a crumble topping.

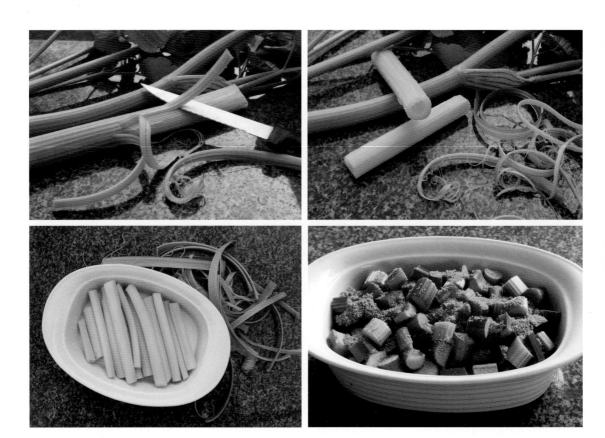

Alexanders **Roots**

Like many wild plants, the flavor of alexanders root is quite variable, with some being much stronger than others. Alexanders is biennial, flowering and seeding in its second year and then dying. The green parts of the first-year plants die back completely in summer when the older plants die, but then emerge again in the autumn or winter when new seedlings also emerge. Roots are best dug in spring, before the older plants start to flower. Winter roots that we have eaten tend to be more bitter and strongly flavored than spring roots.

Golden alexanders (see p14) is a perennial North American relative of alexanders, so its growing pattern differs. It is also edible though some foragers advise against eating its roots.

The roots are whitish cream, with a thin light brown to black skin. The skin can easily be scraped off, but doesn't seem to affect the taste if left on. Remove any whiskery rootlets from the taproot, and scrub them well. We parboil the roots first to reduce any bitterness, before they are sautéed or roasted. The flavor is pleasantly starchy, a bit like parsnip.

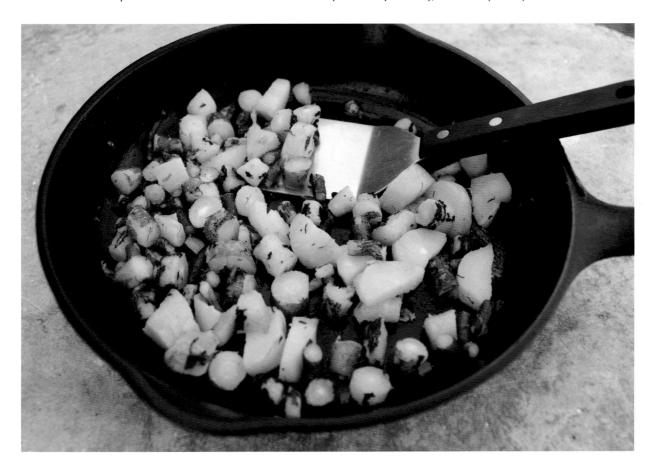

Blackberry

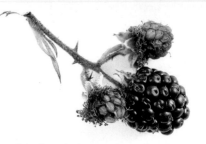

We use the name blackberry (*Rubus fruticosus* agg.) in this book but might have opted for the everyday name bramble. Sometimes for fun we tongue-twistingly combine the words as 'blamble'. It's an aggregate term for an aggregate subject, the king of weeds, whose tasty berries tempt us to put up with its rampant ways. Going brambling is one of the few remaining communal or family foraging activities that draw us into the wild.

**Rosaceae
Rose family**

Perennial.

Edible parts: The ripe fruit in late summer; young shoots anytime but mainly in spring; leaves for tea, mainly in summer.

Distinguishing features: One of the easier wild weeds to identify: universally common, forming an impenetrable rambling, thorny bush with white/pink flowers, then fruit that turns from green to red to black (often all on the same stem at once); rough, mostly evergreen leaves and notorious curved spines that have injured many a gardener or gatherer.

Similar related edible species: Dewberry (*Rubus caesius*) is less common but has blackberry-like fruit with fewer and larger drupelets with a bluish-black bloom; deciduous wild raspberry (*R. idaeus*) has sweet red berries in summer.

Caution: The only caution is to avoid injury from the spines while picking.

What kind of a weed is blackberry?

There are one-word answers to this question. We like rumbustious (British) or rambunctious (American), but can easily add unstoppable, fierce, adaptable, hardy, remarkable …

Blackberry is arguably the king of weeds. Consider its many survival attributes, its essential weedness:

1. Blackberry is actually not a single wild species; botanically, it is an aggregate of over 330 microspecies.

These are so challenging to tell apart, even with microscopes, that blackberry geeks – these people do exist – have their own word for what they do: batology (from old Greek *baton*, for blackberry).

Luckily you don't have to be a batologist because for practical purposes all the *Rubus* species are safe and tasty to eat and use.

2. In addition to normal sexual reproduction, blackberry infant plants can develop asexually. Small, random mutations are sometimes passed on unchanged (the process is called apomixis) into plants that are slightly different; these are the microspecies.

Rubus types, including raspberry, are able to switch between apomictic and sexual reproductive methods as the environment dictates.

3. *Rubus* also displays rampant hybridization, evident in modern crossed commercial varieties like tayberry, boysenberry and youngberry, as well as the older loganberry.

4. The fruit is 'pippy', with sturdy seeds that can pass through the stomach unharmed, whether of a bird, a wild animal or your own, thus spreading far and wide.

5. The fruit will ripen even in the rain.

6. Seed production is prolific: one elmleaf blackberry (*R. ulmifolius*) studied over several years produced 170,000 seeds in a poor year and 400,000 in a favorable one.

7. Seed survival time is long, with a seed bank of up to a hundred years.

8. First-year growth sees the young stems (canes) spreading vigorously, up to 10cm (4.5in) of growth a week in optimal conditions. The thin, light green spears sometimes arch through and over foliage nearby.

In our garden we observed one such spear, which reached 6m (20ft) before it landed. Who says there are no lianas in temperate Europe?

9. When the tip reaches ground it transforms from shoot to root, and starts a new base for future spreading. Unchecked, the result is thickets of dominant blackberry colonies.

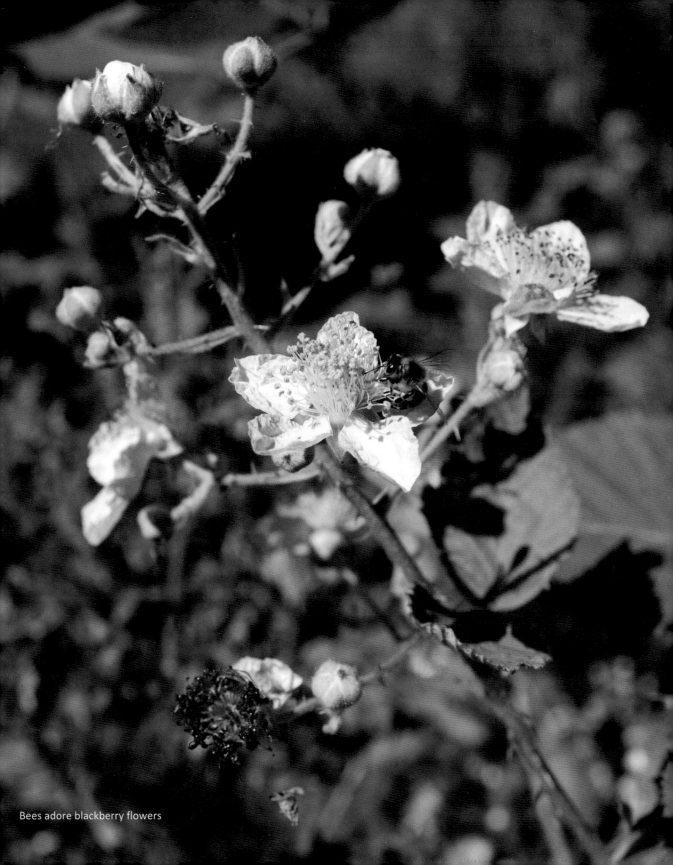

Bees adore blackberry flowers

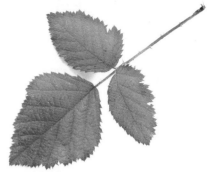

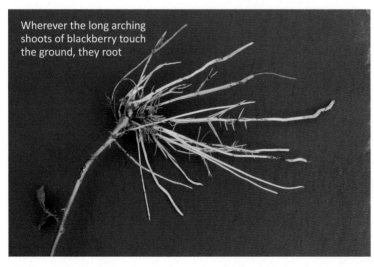

Wherever the long arching shoots of blackberry touch the ground, they root

10. Meanwhile underground the original roots spread widely and go deep. New shoot growth also takes place from the central roots.

11. White or pink blackberry flowers – the only soft thing about this ferocious plant – usually arise in the second year, while leaves can remain evergreen in mild winters. In our local (deciduous) wood blackberry is the prevalent green growth over winter.

12. *Rubus* flourishes in most soil types, and survives assaults by snow, frost, rain, heat, wind and drought.

13. Blackberry is highly competitive in accessing water, nutrients and light. It grows quickly, has a long active season and tolerates low light by extending its leaf area, so thriving in woodland habitats as well as open fields or gardens.

14. At any one time the flowers can appear alongside green, unripe fruit, red ripening fruit and black ready-to-pick fruit on the same stem (p28).

15. The plant's defence mechanism of sharp, backward-pointing spines also helps it be offensive. Around the world blackberry makes an impressive hedge to keep stock or people either in or out.

16. The spines assist growing shoots to force a way through competing foliage, but they cannot be withdrawn easily or painlessly, as we can all testify.

Punctured skin, black-colored hands, and nicks or cuts on the arms and legs are the price we pay for the free food that ripe blackberries offer.

17. Finally, look at the company blackberry keeps. Sometimes called a 'native invasive' and a 'thug' species, in Europe it chooses gangster companions like nettles, ivy, bracken and dog's mercury.

Given half a chance each of these invasives becomes dominant in its locality, while together they create an impenetrable wilderness in the garden.

The history of blackberry
Most of the history of blackberry is unwritten, and early recorded uses of it from Greece, India, China and other ancient cultures are usually medicinal – it is a universal astringent tea for mouth and digestive issues and diarrhea – rather than gustatory.

No doubt people have always taken advantage of blackberry's generous fruiting habit – think how welcome as free food it must be in barren mountainous or tundra areas.

There is no certainty about its place of origin, though the Caucasus has its advocates. Blackberry's travel around the northern hemisphere was effected millennia ago, and in North America some species may have arrived via the Alaskan land-bridge and proceeded to hybridize with native *Rubus* forms.

Blackberry's journey into the southern hemisphere is altogether more recent.

Its colonization followed the European settlers, roughly the 16th century in South America, 17th century in southern Africa, 18th century in Australia and 19th century in New Zealand.

Everywhere it went, blackberry aggressively took over disturbed or post-fire land, whether neglected or cultivated. It not only invaded the wild but it became the wild. It was foragable food for humans and deer (especially roe deer).

And it left evidence of ancient presence if not of human use. In many archaeological sites blackberry seeds abound, with a recognizable diamond-pane window or triangular pattern; the equally well-distributed raspberry seed is larger and rounder.

Because it was universal and familiar as a wild plant and weed blackberry was not grown in gardens or as a crop until modern times.

In the 19th century blackberry was seen as a potential food crop and efforts at hybridization began, culminating in many hybrid edible forms. In Eastern Europe, an important current production area, commercial gathering is still largely from the wild.

Herbal & other uses of blackberry

One historic use is in **basket weaving**. We have tried this ourselves, using freshly cut thin canes (no thicker than a pencil, we were told by our tutor).

The canes are used fresh but their spines must first be removed, using stout gauntlets. The canes are a flexible weaving material that dries to a resilient final shape.

A variant is the woven structures called skeps, made from straw or reeds and bound together by blackberry stems. These were an old style of **beehive**.

In **thatching** twists of blackberry canes were sometimes employed to tie the bundles to the roof; these were known as bands or bonds.

Blackberry fruits and shoots gave a **black dye**, but this was not fast and soon decayed to a sludgy pink. The roots could yield an orange dye of equal impermanency.

In her acclaimed book on wilding at Knepp in Sussex, Isabella Tree (2018) points out the importance of pioneer thorn scrub (*Rubus*) species in a **developing wild ecosystem**, with blackberry alongside hawthorn, blackthorn and wild rose.

She emphasizes that scrub is not wasteland. Far from it: *emerging scrub is one of the richest natural habitats on the planet*. Nightingales, a threatened bird species, are now abundant in Knepp's scrubland. Many other birds, mammals and insects are thankful for the blackberry-rich wildland there.

In **medicinal terms**, one survey of Western herbalism (Tobyn et al., 2011) found, blackberry is unusual in its

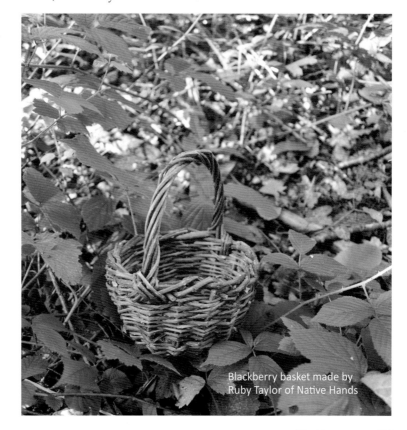

Blackberry basket made by Ruby Taylor of Native Hands

unbroken tradition of similar use over millennia. Much of what Dioscorides (died cAD90) and Pliny the Elder (d. AD 79) recommended for the plant remains current and still practiced today.

For example, Dioscorides said chewing blackberry leaves strengthens the gums. He noted how blackberry contracts and dries the tissues, a feature we now call astringency, based on the tannic, malic and citric acids.

American herbal writer Maida Silverman (1997) summarizes: *It is difficult to overestimate the faith people once had in the healing powers of this plant.* The astringency, she notes, is present through all parts – leaves, roots, flowers, ripe and unripe berries.

Eating the young shoots, cooked as a tender vegetable or pounded into a juice in a mortar and pestle, following Pliny, was thought to fasten loose teeth in the gums and treat diarrhea and dysentery.

Blackberry tea is another suggestion by Pliny. Whether for mouth ulcers, quinsy (a form of tonsillitis), stomach upsets, upset menstruation, cystitis or hemorrhoids, a blackberry tea or gargle remains a safe treatment.

We would now say the effectiveness of blackberry is not only that it is rich in minerals and vitamins but that these are readily bio-available and well absorbed.

Externally, blackberry tea is an excellent hair rinse after shampooing, though as a black hair dye it is only effective short-term. Use the cooled tea too as a lotion for sunburn and minor burns.

There are no cautions against using blackberries medicinally, though (as many foragers know) eating too many at once while you gather is inevitable and may result in a cramped stomach.

How to eat blackberry

How do you tell if a blackberry is good to eat? A way we have learned is to check the heel (or hilum) when you pull the fruit body off. If the hilum is dark or messy there will probably be an insect within; if it is white or pale green, no insect.

When picking, beware the spines, and don't pack the fruit too deep in your basket. The fruit is surprisingly squishy and the lower layers may turn to liquid.

Blackberry syrups, jams or wine are appetizing ways to take your blackberry medicine internally, while a vinegar might be helpful against fevers. The berries can be fermented into a wine or a beer.

The ripe black berries are used for bramble jam; for best results in making bramble jelly some of the red half-ripe ones are added for their pectin content.

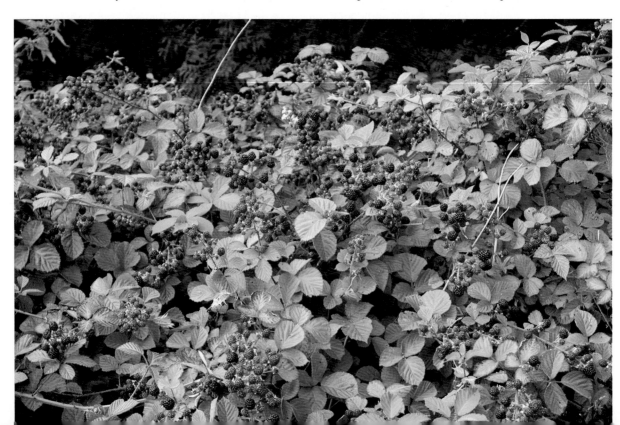

Blackberry with **Pancakes**

Cook fresh blackberries lightly with some sugar to make the perfect topping for fluffy American-style breakfast pancakes. Frozen blackberries can also be used, but the juices might need to cook a bit longer to thicken. Makes 6 pancakes.

For the pancakes, mix **150g (1¼ cups) spelt or wheat flour** with **37g (¼ cup) gram flour** (or chickpea/garbanzo flour), **2 teaspoons baking powder, 2 tablespoons demerara sugar** and **½ teaspoon salt**. Stir in **250ml (1 cup) water, 1 teaspoon vinegar** and **2 tablespoons vegetable oil**, just until mixed.

Pour spoonfuls of batter into a hot, lightly oiled skillet to make 10–12cm (4- or 5-in) pancakes. When bubbles have come to the surface and broken, and the pancake is set around the edges, turn the pancake over and cook the other side until golden. Keep the pancakes warm while you cook the rest of the batter.

Heat **a couple of cups of blackberries** in a saucepan with **a little sugar (2 to 4 tablespoons of light brown sugar or coconut nectar sugar)**. Cook for just long enough for the juice to come out of the blackberries and thicken into a syrup.

Serve a stack of pancakes with the blackberry mixture poured over the top.

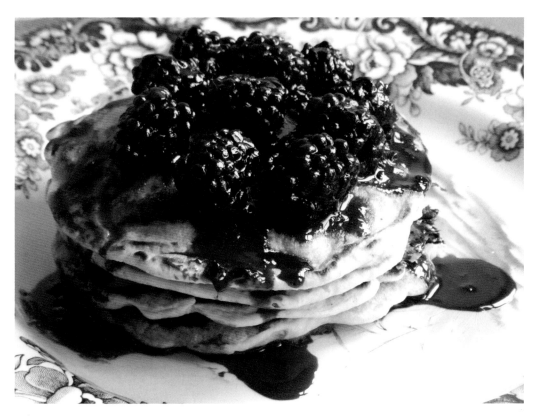

Blackberry **Butter**

This recipe combines blackberries with apples to give a lovely thick spread that is delicious on bread or toast.

The proportion of apples to blackberries is up to you, but anywhere from a third to a half blackberries will give a lovely rich color.

Wash the fruit, and coarsely chop the apples. They don't need to be peeled or cored. Weigh the fruit and see how many lemons you will need: for each 1kg (2¼ lb) of your fruit (**blackberries and apples**) you will need **the juice and finely grated zest of a lemon.** Put the fruit in a saucepan with the lemon zest and juice. Simmer gently for about 15 minutes or until the fruit is soft and mushy.

Push the fruit through a sieve to remove skins and seeds.

Weigh the sieved fruit pulp, and you will need about half the weight in **sugar**. Adjust the sweetness to the sweetness of the fruit, and your taste.

Heat the fruit pulp and sugar gently until the sugar dissolves, and continue cooking gently while stirring to make a smooth, thick creamy mixture. This will probably take about 20 minutes.

Pour into warm sterilized jars and seal. Label. Will keep just like jam, but refrigerate once it has been opened.

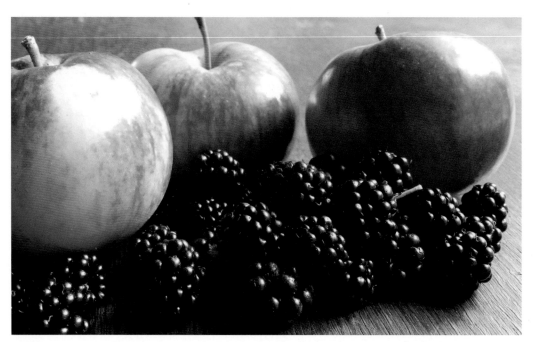

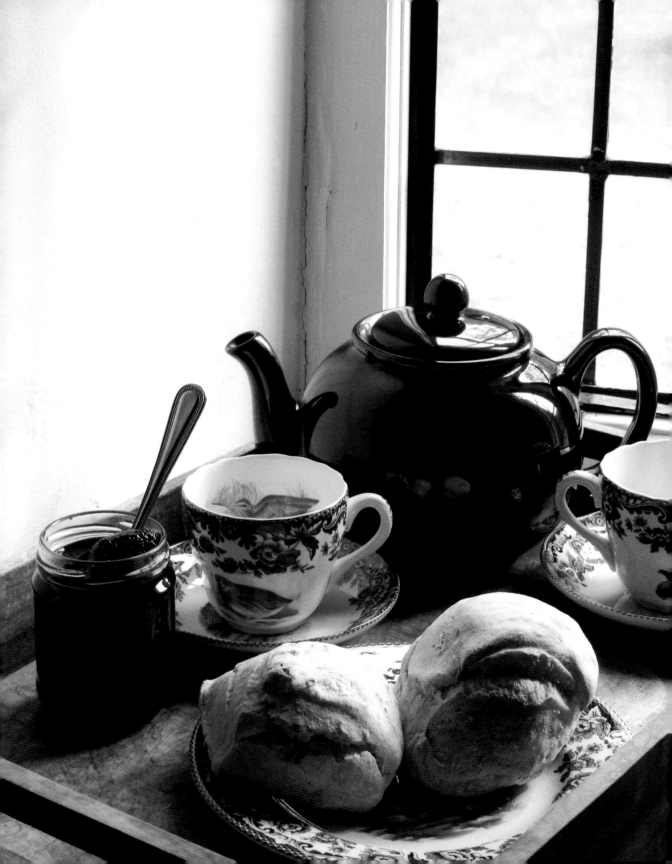

Blackberry **Flummery**

This recipe came from Julie's grandmother, and is probably over a hundred years old. Flummeries were popular from the 17th century, and evolved from an oatmeal-based pudding to any soft-set pudding. In Sydney Julie's mother used to earn pocket money by collecting blackberries, which are an invasive species in Australia.

Wash **4 cups blackberries**
Combine in a saucepan with   **125ml (½ cup) hot water**
    250g (1¼ cups) sugar
Add **a dash of salt and cinnamon**.

Bring mixture to a boiling point, reduce heat and simmer until slightly syrupy – about 5 to 8 minutes.

Mix   **3 tablespoons water**
    2 tablespoons cornstarch until a smooth paste is formed.

Blend this mixture into the hot blackberry mixture. Stir while cooking until the mixture is thickened and slightly translucent – about 3 to 5 minutes.

Pour into a serving bowl. Cool and serve cold.

Serves 6.

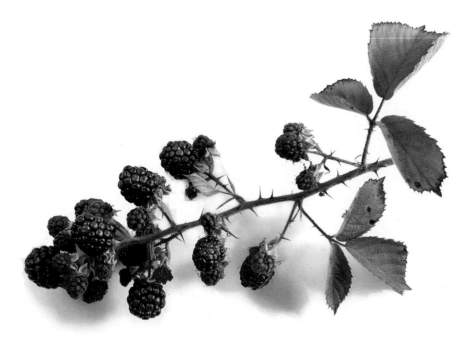

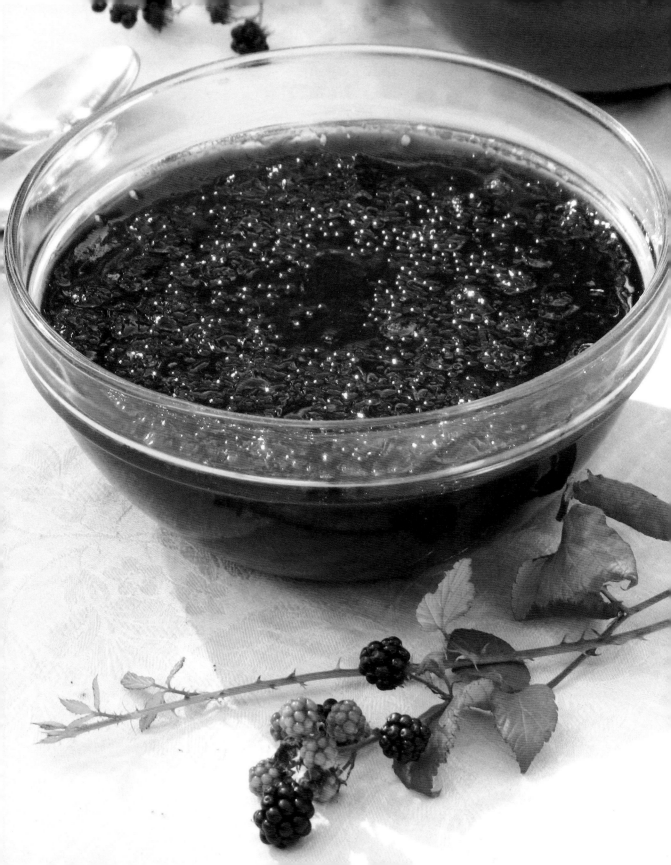

Blackberry Passionfruit **Pavlova**

Passionfruit and blackberries are the perfect complement to light, airy meringue and coconut cream. Our meringue is made with aqua faba (bean water) instead of egg whites. Chickpeas (garbanzos) are the most common source of aqua faba, but the liquid from cooked or tinned borlotti beans and other beans can also be used. Red kidney bean water gives a pretty, pale pink meringue. Aqua faba is sometimes also available to buy as an egg substitute. Use aqua faba at room temperature for best results.

To make the meringue: In an electric mixer, beat **aqua faba from a tin of chickpeas** until stiff peaks form – usually 10 to 15 minutes.
Add **¼ teaspoon cream of tartar**.
Slowly add **200g (1 cup) golden caster sugar (baker's or superfine sugar)**, a little at a time
The mixture should be thick and glossy.

Pipe onto baking paper in a circle or circles, with an extra layer around the rim. You can make a big pavlova or individual smaller ones, and any extra meringue mixture can be made into small meringues.

The meringue needs to be baked at a low temperature for a long time. If the oven is too hot, the meringue will go flat and brown. Bake at 120C/250F until dry and crisp on the outside – the time depends on the size of your pavlovas and the humidity, but allow an hour or more. Allow to cool slowly.

Top with **whipped coconut cream** or **thick coconut yogurt**. To make the passionfruit to go on top, mix **the pulp of two or three passionfruit** with **2 to 3 tablespoons of icing sugar**.

Spread the passionfruit over the cream layer, and top with **lots of fresh blackberries**.

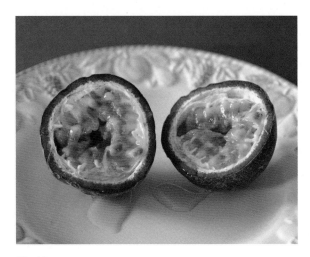 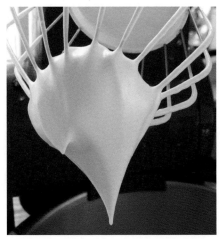

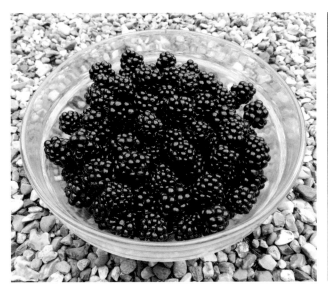

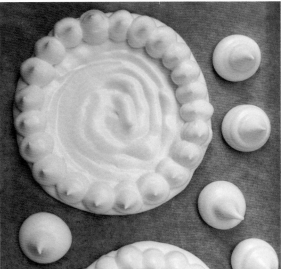

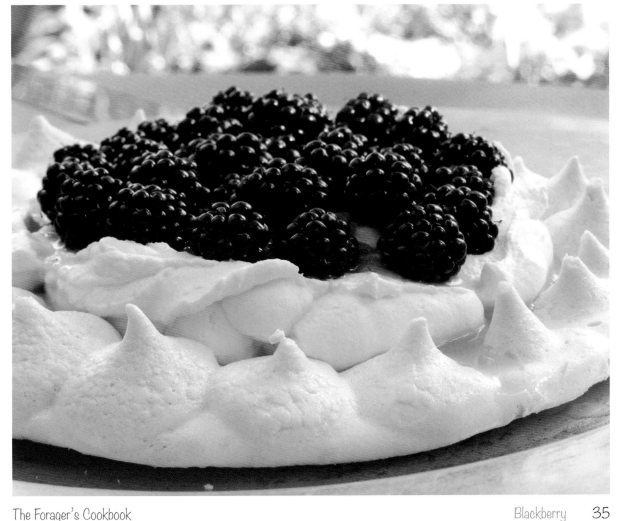

Blackberry & Plum Jam

This is a really quick and easy recipe for a delicious jam that isn't too sweet. We prefer jam sugar, which has added pectin, because then we can use less sugar overall and still get a good set. Heating the sugar stops it from cooling the fruit mixture.

You can use more sugar if you like a sweeter jam or want to preserve it for longer. Here we foraged wild golden cherry plums that were ripe at the same time as our blackberries.

Pit the **plums** and weigh them with the **blackberries**. Put them in a pan and heat until the juice starts to flow.

You will need half the weight of your fruit in **jam sugar**. Heat it by spreading on a tray in the oven. Don't heat it for too long or it will caramelize.

Add the hot sugar to the cooking fruit and heat rapidly for 8 to 12 minutes, which preserves the fresh taste of the fruit. If you have a jam thermometer you can check it's nearing the jam setting point of 105C/220F; otherwise just test a little on a cold saucer to see if it's setting.

Pour into clean hot jars and seal. Best kept in a cool place. Refrigerate once opened.

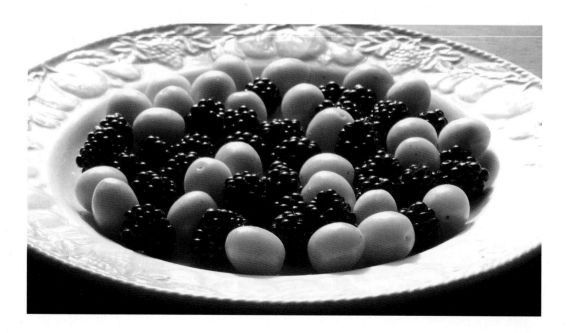

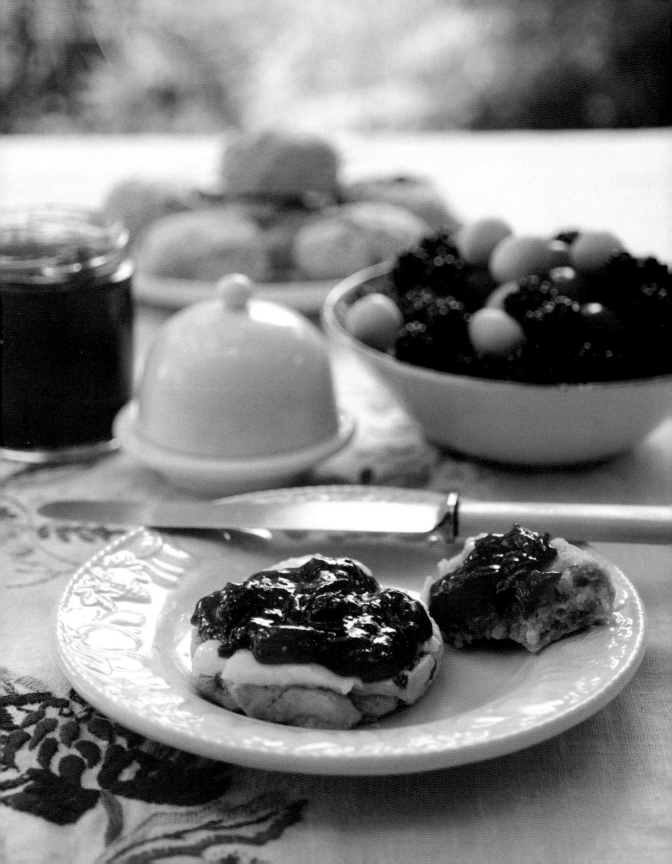

Chickweed

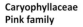

Chickweed (*Stellaria media*) is an example of good things coming in small bundles. Both as food and medicine it is a powerhouse whose unappreciated benefits would astonish the gardener who despairs of eliminating this cheery, bright green plant. An American forager calls it a blessing for those suffering from winter F.W.S. (Forager's Withdrawal Syndrome). Here is your invitation to get your chickweed chloro-fill!

**Caryophyllaceae
Pink family**

Annual or short-lived perennial. Prefers cool, moist conditions.

Edible parts: All above-ground parts, gathered whenever vibrant and green, mainly in spring and autumn.

Distinguishing features: A sprawling annual plant to about 15cm (6in) high, with lime green leaves and tiny star-like white flowers. The stem is rounded and hairless, apart from the special feature of a line of small white hairs running up one side, then alternating to the other side after a leaf node. Sometimes the hairs are on both sides.

Caution: The main caution is for harvesting, to make sure you are not including spurge with your chickweed (see p41). Avoid eating very large amounts of chickweed because of the saponin content.

What kind of a weed is chickweed?

Chickweed is *stellaria*, a star, with, as one herbalist puts it, *as glamorous a name as any prima donna*. This refers to the five-pointed green star of the calyx holding the pretty white starburst of a flower with its tiny reddish anthers.

Its other Latin name is more prosaic, *media* or middle, for its place between two less common European species, greater chickweed (*Stellaria neglecta*) and lesser chickweed (*S. pallida*).

The common name has old forms, like chick wittles, clucken wort and chickeny weed, which confirm chickweed as a fowl favorite. This can be attested worldwide: giving personal references, the young Julie gathered chickweed for her grandmother's chickens in Australia, and Matthew's mother in Cambridgeshire fed her caged canaries on fresh chickweed flowers and seeds. But neither lady was known to try the taste themselves.

Why should birds have all the fun? Chickweed is an excellent salad plant for us too, especially in late winter and early spring, when there's little else

green and fresh available for foraging. This is literally a winter-green!

Chickweed is indeed available almost all year round, in most cool temperate climates. In midsummer it doesn't like hot dry weather, but may be found in moist shady spots, and in mid-winter it disappears in colder climes.

We might call it almost a genteel weed, though gardeners will not agree. It is its habit of springing up quickly on bare earth and forming a dense cover that potentially can starve or shade other seedlings that makes it an old enemy.

But, if you don't like it, it is easily pulled up, with little resistance; moreover from a gardening point of view its presence signals fertile soil and it helps keep the soil moist. We suggest that once you agree how good it is, for food and medicine, you'll never seem to have enough of it.

The universality of chickweed can be accounted for by its rapid reproduction rate. This is described well in Sir Edward Salisbury's 1961 survey, *Weeds & Aliens*. A classic of the 'identify weeds and then destroy them by

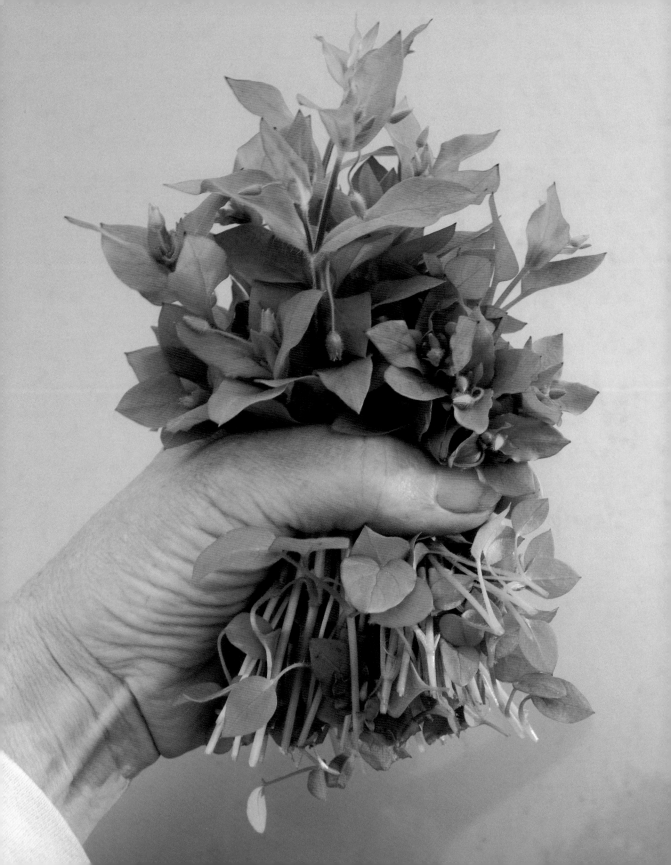

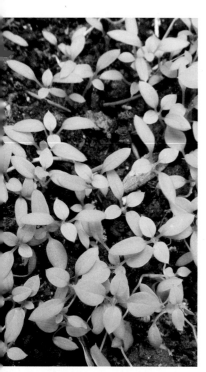

Chickweed seedlings can be picked and eaten as micro-greens, or left to grow bigger.

chemicals' school, the book is still a presence in modern weed lore.

What Sir Edward explains is how chickweed seeds germinate almost as soon as they hit the ground, and given favorable moist conditions the entire life cycle from seed to seed can be accomplished in 5 to 7 weeks. Because the flowering season is not governed by day length, individual plants can bloom at more or less any time.

One plant can put out 2,500 seeds, and there might be three generations a year. If most of these were to survive, over a year there could be over 15,000 million plants. Sir Edward estimates these might cover an area the size of the Isle of Wight three times. For North American readers, think roughly the area of Las Vegas, then triple it.

Add to this that the seeds can be viable for 25 years, and perhaps 40, and that cold weather is not a barrier, and you can appreciate how chickweed survives Ice Ages, life in the Arctic Circle and the bare patches in our own gardens. The only surprise is that has not yet achieved world domination.

The history of chickweed

The oldest record we have come across is of preserved chickweed pollen identified at a site in Hoxne, Suffolk, with a calibrated date of about 400,000 years ago. No doubt our ancestors then were grateful for it as food rather than condemning the plant as a weed.

This was during an interglacial period, and many chickweed Ice Age occurrences are known. Closer to our own time, in the early 1950s, the 'bog bodies' in Denmark, known as Tollund man and Grauballe man, dating to some 2,400 years ago, had numerous wild plant remains in their stomachs.

Their full bellies probably reflect an elaborate ritual meal, and one ingredient was seed of *Stellaria media*, along with chickweed's meadow cousin, *Spergula arvensis*, corn spurrey.

Chickweed seed survives passage through an animal or a bird's gut, and even immersion in seawater. In Iceland, for example, it spreads in sheep droppings. This toughness helps explain its spread and survival from a Eurasian origin to straddle the world.

Greeks and Romans of the classical period grew chickweed as a crop as well as wild-gathering it for food and for making cooling poultices.

Chickweed is part of a rice porridge dish prepared for the spring festival in Japan, dating from the 9th century. The celebration still continues each year on 7 January, as *Nanak no sekku*, the Festival of Seven Herbs.

The seven prized plants varied locally but typically consisted of young leaves or roots of Java water dropwort or parsley (this species is safe to eat, unlike the European hemlock water dropwort, which is poisonous), shepherd's purse, cudweed, chickweed, nipplewort, turnip and radish.

The chickweed family has always been 'winter-green', and it is no surprise that the succulent sea chickweed (*Honckenya peploides*) is found north of the Arctic Circle. There it is pickled by the Innuit (Eskimos), as the only green vegetable in their almost exclusively animal-based diet.

Herbal & other uses of chickweed

If condensing chickweed's herbal attributes into a single word, 'nourishment' would be a good candidate. Whether outwardly or inwardly, chickweed supports, moistens, protects and nourishes.

Its best-known external use is to soothe itches, bites, stings, inflammations, burns, swellings, sunburn, bruises, splinters and sore eyes. It makes a good and readily found first-aid or emergency remedy – simply pull up a handful and place directly onto the affected part. If you have more time, crush some chickweed with a mortar and pestle, and bandage the paste across the wound or bite as a poultice. This treatment is also cooling and soothing for sunburn.

Chickweed has the particular reputation of resolving skin problems where some form of heat is involved and where other herbs or creams have failed, especially when a cooling, drawing action is needed.

It is useful to alleviate long-standing or 'indolent' issues, such as eczema, rheumatic joints and varicose veins.

Chickweed contains plentiful saponins. Saponin means 'soap-like' – a related plant is soapwort (*Saponaria officinalis*).

If you take a handful of chickweed and rub it in your hands with a little water, you may not actually get a lather, but you'll feel the soapiness and it'll leave your hands feeling pampered and soft, with just a faint smell of the plant.

Saponins work at a cellular level to increase absorption and permeability. What this means is that inflamed organ membranes, as in the liver, kidneys and lungs, are helped by saponins to absorb healing nutrients, as well as allowing their wastes and blockages to be more easily removed. Add to this the cooling qualities of chickweed, and you have a wonderful, subtle herbal cleanser and restorer at work, rather than the usual dismissive mention in modern herbals of using it for 'itchiness'.

It also has reputed value as a slimming aid. Chickweed water or tea is a folk remedy for the overweight, and dried chickweed is found in some proprietary slimming formulas.

Some herbalists believe it does work, as the saponins help to dissolve body fat; others note it stimulates urination, so will assist in shedding body moisture, which would contribute to weight loss. As with many treatments, what is effective for one may not be so for all.

Very large amounts of saponins can potentially be toxic, causing digestive upsets, so don't overdo it, but eating normal amounts is fine.

Overall chickweed has a valuable toning action for the body's internal organs. In American herbalist Susun Weed's words, it 'sponges up the spills' and 'tidies up the rips'. She cites the plant's 'deep mending skills', and how it relieves, clears, protects and nourishes.

Whether as a salad, tea or tincture, poultice or vinegar, chickweed is effective, available, free and safe.

How to harvest and eat chickweed

Gathering your chickweed harvest is simplicity itself. Start with the right mental approach: look at the chickweed bed as a field of microgreens, and think you are harvesting, not weeding.

Cut off the top inch or two of the young plants with scissors (pulling will uproot them and leave you with another job of snipping off the roots). You can gather a meal in 20 seconds. Your harvest is ready to use as a tender green in a broth, salad or smoothie, and the shorn stems will grow back again.

Pick it over to see that you are not including other small plants, particularly spurge, which often grows among chickweed and has a caustic milky sap, sometimes used on warts: see right.

Chickweed's taste is of chlorophyll, with an earthy, slightly salty tang. The high vitamin A, B6 and B12, C and D levels, saponins and plentiful minerals, including more iron and potassium than spinach, make chickweed a top spring tonic, alone or in combination.

Chickweed has long been eaten fresh by country people and it was once sold in the streets of London. We grow it in pots to overwinter in the greenhouse and harvest it fresh to mix in salads. By itself it is perhaps an acquired taste, but in recipes it is pleasingly tasty.

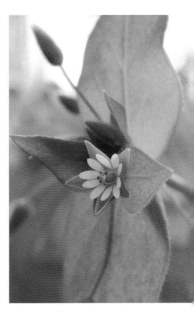

Chickweed has a beautiful star-shaped green calyx holding the white flower. Every flower is made up of 5 petals, but because each one is deeply split it looks like 10.

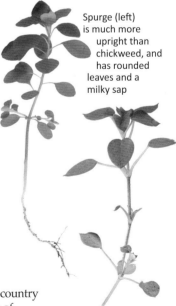

Spurge (left) is much more upright than chickweed, and has rounded leaves and a milky sap

Chickweed is sprawling and floppy, with pointed leaves and clear sap

Chickweed **Pesto**

This is our favorite wild pesto recipe. It's so delicious that we make it at Thanksgiving, at Christmas and whenever we have enough chickweed. It is perfect when you are craving something fresh and green. It goes well with pasta, but we usually serve it like a side sauce with whatever else we are eating – it complements most savory dishes.

Blend together in a food processor:
100g chickweed (a colander full)
2 or 3 cloves garlic
1 or 2 teaspoons vegetable boullion powder
125ml (½ cup) extra virgin olive oil or cold pressed hemp seed oil
150g (½ cup) sunflower seeds or Brazil nut pieces
2 tablespoons yeast flakes (nutritional yeast)
salt to taste

Alternatives:
You can use cleavers or other greens in place of the chickweed, or use a mixture of your favorites. Pumpkin seeds or pine nuts can be used instead of sunflower seeds.

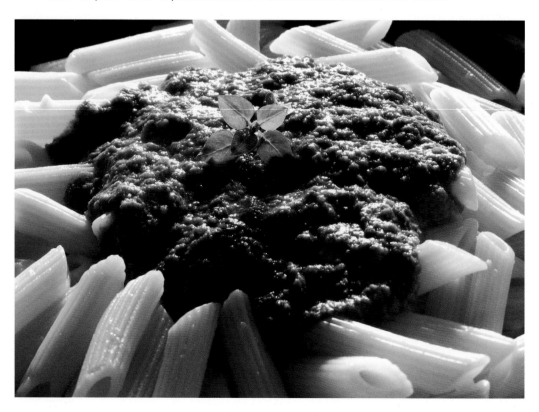

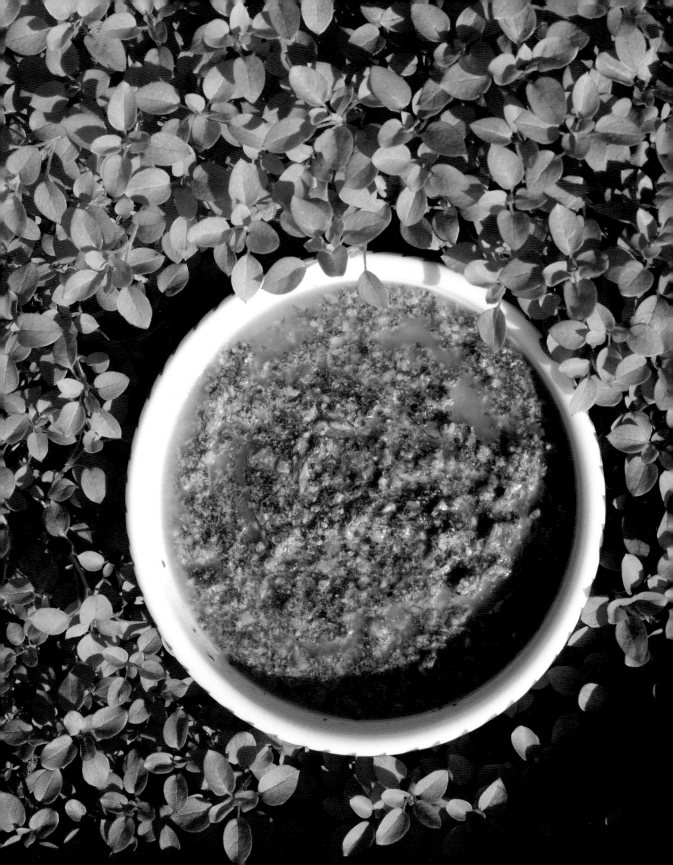

Chickweed & Peach **Salad**

Chickweed is a good addition to any green salad, but looks particularly beautiful in this colorful salad with peaches, raw purple cauliflower, tomato and onion.

Slice **2 ripe peaches, 3 or 4 tomatoes, a purple cauliflower** and **a small onion or shallot**. Take **a double handful of chickweed** and snip off the top inch or so of each sprig to use in the salad – the rest can be saved for pesto or cooking.

Arrange on a large plate. Drizzle with your choice of dressing, or try the recipe opposite.

Alternatives:
If you like extra crunch, try adding toasted slivered almonds or toasted pumpkin seeds.

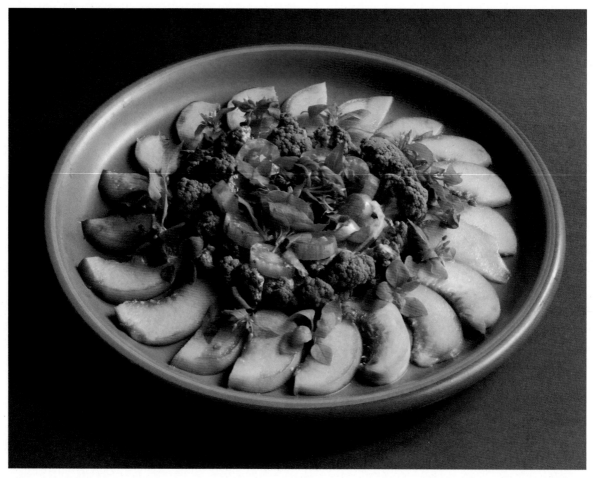

Citrus Dressing for Chickweed & Peach Salad

This citrus-rich dressing goes well with peach salad, but also with cabbage salads as a fresher alternative to mayonnaise and creamy dressings. Put all the ingredients in a jar and shake well. Couldn't be easier!

125ml (½ cup) extra virgin olive oil
2 tablespoons white wine vinegar, or white balsamic vinegar
2 tablespoons fresh orange juice
1 tablespoon finely grated organic orange zest
1 tablespoon lemon or lime juice
1 clove of garlic, minced

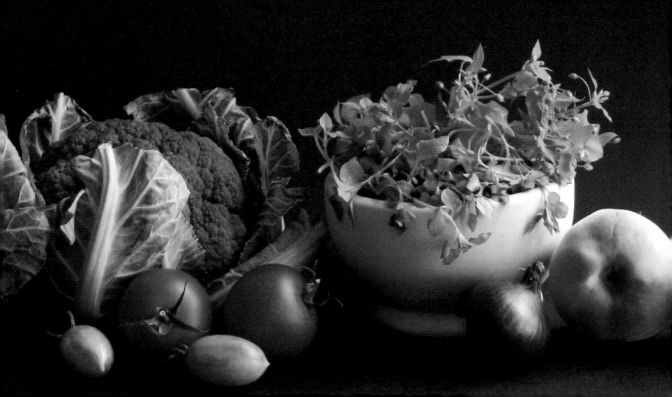

Chickweed **Hummus**

Chickweed gives a lovely pale green color to hummus and increases the nutritional benefits, being a particularly good source of iron – higher even than nettles.

Put in a food processor:
480g (2 cups) cooked chickpeas (garbanzos)
2 cloves garlic
a good double handful of chickweed (about 50g)
juice of half a lemon
1 teaspoon salt or to taste
130g (½ cup) tahini
125ml (½ cup) water, if needed to mix well

It depends how liquid your tahini is and how juicy your chickpeas are, but you will probably need the water to make the mixture wet enough to mix properly. Taste and adjust the seasonings if necessary.

Alternatives: Nutritional yeast flakes add an extra umami savoriness – start by adding a tablespoon.

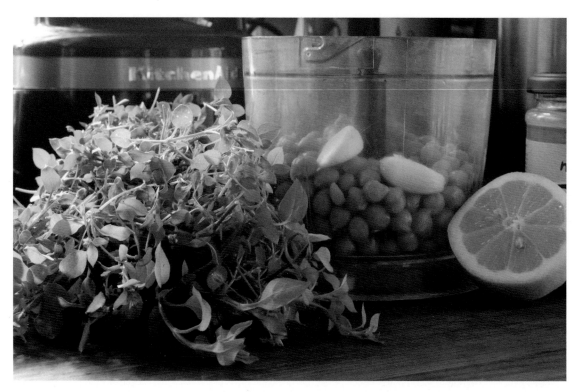

Chickweed **Crostini**

Fry **1 long shallot, diced finely,** and **2 tablespoons pine (or cedar) nuts** in **a little oil**, until translucent.

Rinse **4 good handfuls of chickweed** and chop coarsely (remove stems if stringy).

While still wet, add to the shallot and nuts, then cook gently until wilted and the smell has changed from chickweedy to mild.

Add **salt** and **lemon juice** to taste.

Grill **6 to 8 slices of baguette** both sides and heap the cooked mixture on.

Alternatives: The chickweed mixture is also good with boiled new potatoes.

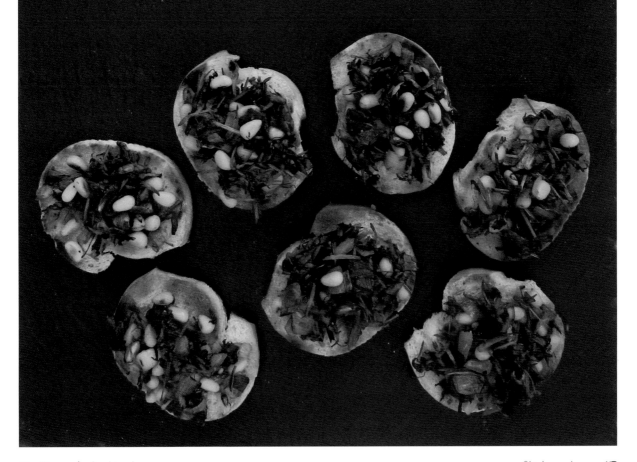

Cleavers

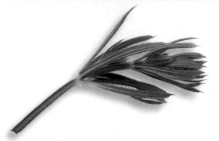

Cleavers, goosegrass or sticky willy (*Galium aparine*) may seem an unlikely source of palatable wild food and drinks recipes. Much too 'scratchy', you might say. But the seedlings in early spring are smoother, and the tiny hooks still soft, yielding a tasty, alkaline freshness and good mineral nutrition that we can take advantage of. Moussaka and stir fry are excellent 'tips', too.

Rubiaceae
Bedstraw (Coffee) family

Annual. Plants germinate in autumn or late winter, and die back after fruiting in late summer.

Edible parts: Young tips, picked from winter through until flowering in early summer. Ripe fruits gathered in summer to roast for coffee.

Distinguishing features: Clambering plant covered in tiny hook-like bristles which help it climb up hedges and other plants, or to stick to your clothes. Leaves are in whorls around the stem. Cleavers has tiny four-petalled white flowers in summer, followed by round hairy fruits in pairs.

Edible relatives: Sweet woodruff, *Galium odoratum*, is prized as a flavoring for drinks.

Caution: The bristles can irritate the skin when weeding – wear long sleeves.

What kind of a weed is cleavers?

We have a strong visual memory of cleavers (*Galium aparine*). Some twenty summers back we were attending an herbal event in Somerset, in England's West Country.

In a country lane near our destination we had to stop the car for a second look. In a section of hedgerow, some 3m (10ft) high and at least 30m (100ft) long, all the hawthorns, maples and wild roses were covered, top to bottom, with a lime-green filigree of cleavers.

It was as if a living green shawl had been thrown over the hedge. Here was cleavers trumpeting its unchecked vigor and essence – its *viriditas*, in the term used by Hildegard of Bingen, the 12th-century German abbess, composer and herbalist.

This demonstration of the speed at which cleavers can spread is well attested in descriptive English country names like robin run by the dyke and lizzie run the hedge.

A friend of ours teaches survival skills to airmen. He described the almost universal failure of his students, once taken into the outdoors, to see individual species of plants.

They experience a 'green wall', he said, and his challenge was to open the airmen's eyes to the diversity and potential of forageable and medicinal plants that might save their lives.

Cleavers, though, stands out; it is the quintessential plant that cleaves or grips – 'grip grass' in some localities.

The stems and leaves, and particularly the fruits, readily attach to us, our livestock or pets, just as they do to vegetation, bedding plants or arable crops in hedges, gardens and fields.

This growth habit inspires both 'sticky' names – sticky bob, stickyback and sticky willy – and intimate names – huggy me close, kiss me quick and lover's kisses – where clinging is literal.

Cleavers is an annual, but begins its germination in autumn and early winter. It is one of the first garden weeds to show – a bare and untended raised bed can be filled with hundreds of tiny cleavers plants in a couple of weeks, even with snow on the ground.

These small cleavers, already vigorous, are a bane to the gardener, but a tasty boon of potential freshness to the early-season forager.

Once mature, the stems can be easily pulled away. The Irish naturalist and author Michael Viney (2013) describes weeding his cleavers as like *hauling in a fishing net, as the stems, often three meters long, gather up others as they come: one keeps pulling slowly, hand over hand*.

We agree with Viney about how satisfying this form of weeding is, and also note his addendum, that it is 'only mildly effective' as the stems of the

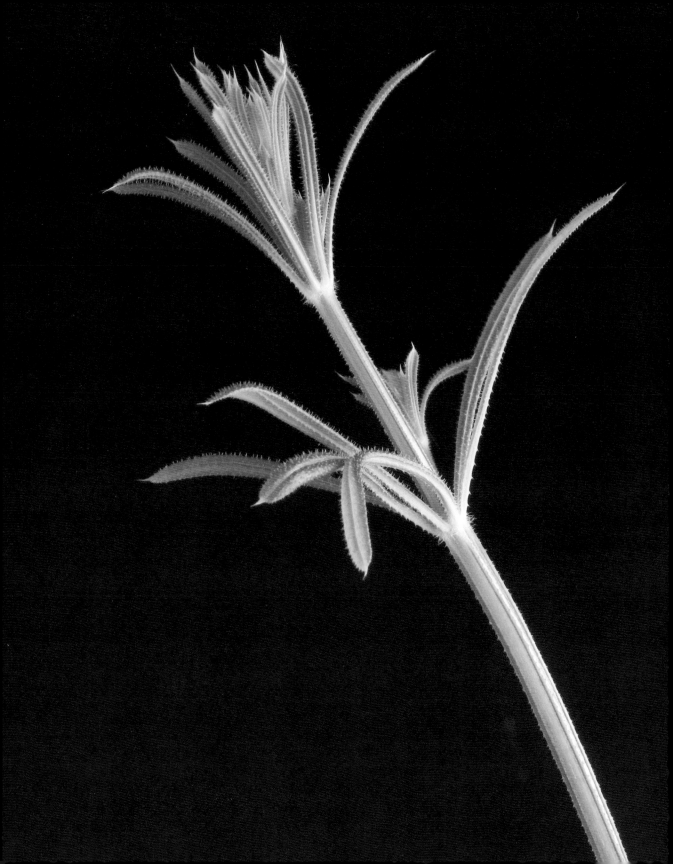

Below: infant cleavers as you are likely to see it in winter (compare with baby chickweed, p41); right: full summer cleavers growth, easily swamping nettle and fruiting wild raspberry

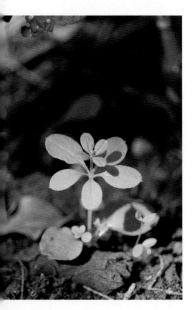

cleavers snap off above the root, which grows back. When weeding, it's best to wear long sleeves as the hooks can irritate the skin, like a carpet burn.

When gathering young cleavers for food, use scissors for a clean cut and to avoid bruising the stems.

In agricultural terms cleavers is generally controllable by farmers but is a notifiable pest of arable crops in parts of North America; in Western Australia, it is a declared pest of canola (rape).

As in many northern hemisphere weeds reaching the south, there are fewer limitations of disease or predation on cleavers' ability to become locally dominant.

Finally, one is known by the company one keeps, and cleavers runs with a racy crowd, including nettle and blackberry. It clambers over them too.

The history of cleavers

The archaeological record for cleavers is patchy, and although its fruits and carbonized seeds are often found in European prehistoric sites, little significance has been given to them.

One exception is the recent discovery of remnants of colored cloth dated to about 2000 years ago in the eastern US. The red dye used was from the roots of local cleavers plants.

This tells us something about Amerindian peoples at that place and time but also supports the contention that cleavers is a native North American plant.

The first US record, reflecting settler culture, was not until John Josselyn's herbal of 1672, where he noted cleavers' presence in New England. Whether that cleavers was of native stock or brought in by settlers is moot.

It is in the Old World that cleavers made its name. Some 2,200 years ago, in his *Enquiry into Plants*, the Greek scholar Theophrastus wrote: *Bedstraw has the peculiarity that it sticks to clothes owing to its roughness, and it is hard to pull away* [translation by Hort, 1916].

Theophrastus used the Greek term *aparo*, clinging or seizing, and this name has 'stuck' in the name *aparine*.

The genus name *Galium* was conferred by the herbal authority Dioscorides about 200 years later, referencing the Greek term for milk. His mentioned how Greek shepherds made small nests of cleavers, bending the stems to create a sieve for filtering animal hairs from fresh milk.

We have also made use of cleaver's plasticity to form wild containers or bowls, perfect for gathering berries.

In the herbal literature cleavers is cited as a vegetable rennet to curdle milk, though nettle, ground ivy and the cleavers' relative Lady's bedstraw (*G. verum*) were used more often.

Another common name for cleavers is goosegrass, and this can be read literally. Geese, especially goslings, love eating the plant, as do other farmyard animals.

There was once a persistent view that cleavers was weak, a feeble dependant on other plants. Two herbal commentators writing a century apart, Pierpoint Johnson (English) in 1862, and Euell Gibbons (American) in 1966, agreed on this.

But in recent years bioengineering research, including 3-D laser examination, has shown that cleavers' spines differ on the upper (adaxial) and lower (abaxial) sides, being arrayed in opposite directions.

The lower hooks provide strong adhesion to adjacent plants, while the upper ones slide off easily. The resulting ratchet mechanism enables clinging or rapid growth as needed.

This is seen especially in cleavers' fruits: for distribution they need to cling easily to the unwary passing person or animal while also detaching readily and not pulling the parent plant apart.

Other research (Goodman 2004) shows that cleavers' square stems have the highest breaking strains of any terrestrial plant so far tested.

Strength and flexibility, and the ability to both grasp and to release, make for appealing biomechanical characteristics.

Possibly cleavers could become as significant an inspiration as burdock (*Arctium lappa*), whose pesky burs catching in his dog's coat so piqued the imagination of one Swiss scientist that he manufactured the hook arrangement as a strong but quick-release strip, and called it Velcro.

Herbal & other uses of cleavers

Cleavers was once a traditional spring tonic herb, as graphically expressed by William Coles in 1656: *for cleansing the blood, strengthening the liver … fitting the Body for the season that follows, by purging away those excrementitious dregs which the Winter has bred in them.*

Culpeper (1652) agreed with the purpose and added the method: the plant is *chopped small and boiled well in water-gruel.*

Peas, beans, onions and other dried, over-wintered foods would be supplemented by cleavers, nettles and other spring weeds as part of cleansing Lenten pottages (i.e. soups or stews).

This quality of mild cleansing is borne out by modern uses of cleavers as a lymphatic herb. It promotes flow in the lymphatic vessels while also ridding them of waste, in effect acting like a pipe cleaner for the lymphatic system.

The conditions that have been treated historically include swollen glands, goitre, tonsillitis and adenoid problems, and earache.

Cleavers has a persistent tradition, now being explored seriously in the laboratory, of being able to shrink tumors and remove nodular growths on the skin, including scrofula (once called 'king's evil' because it was healed, in the popular imagination, by the monarch's touch).

Scrofula is now called mycobacterial (or tuberculous) cervical lymphadenitis.

In the past cleavers was used as a liver herb, capable of treating jaundice without causing liver irritation.

… this study has shown that, in cleavers, the lower stem is highly extensible; breaking strains of approx. 24% were recorded. No other terrestrial plants have been shown to have such extensible stems.
– Goodman (2004)

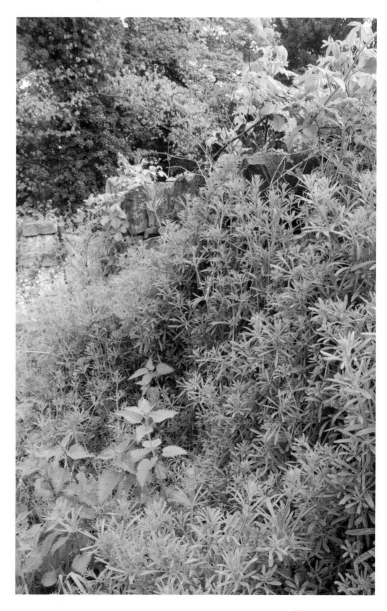

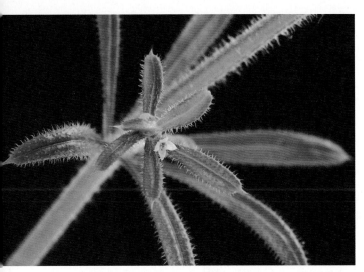

Above: a minute flower of cleavers arising among girder-like green architecture; below right: close-up of the unripe seed balls

Modern herbalists know cleavers as a diuretic, or promoter of the flow of urine. It has a cooling action, gently reducing heat and inflammation in the urinary tract. It is an ingredient in herbal cystitis formulas and for urethritis, irritable bladder, prostatitis and strangury (painful blockage of the bladder).

In its 'pipe cleaner' role cleavers was also used to flush out small calcium deposits, the so-called grit and gravel, from the kidneys and urinary tract.

Cleavers tea is sometimes recommended as an evening drink for sleep. Mrs Grieve (1931) writes that cleavers *has a most soothing effect in cases of insomnia, and induces quiet, restful sleep.* On the other hand, in some people night-time diuretic effects will follow.

The tea, simply heated up and cooled, also makes a home deodorant and can be applied direct or as a poultice to the skin for sunburn, itches, irritations and psoriasis. A paste or ointment made from cleavers is a traditional but also contemporary treatment for leg ulcers.

One more application, known to the ancient Greeks and repeated in later herbals, was cleavers for weight loss.

Back in the garden, your cleavers tangle is an indicator of fertile soil, and a good accumulator of sodium, silica and calcium for a liquid fertilizer or feed. But beware putting your mature cleavers haul on the compost heap: this offers a fertile seedbed for cleavers infants.

The root was once a dye, as mentioned, and another now-forgotten use of cleavers is literally as a bedstraw, as in the family name. The massed stems you weed out in summer could alternatively be used to stuff mattresses, bolsters or pillows at no cost. There is exceptional adhesion and flexibility in the cleavers mass, making a more comfortable natural bed when camping than scratchier bracken or heather.

A near relative of cleavers, the yellow-flowered Lady's bedstraw, was believed to have been used as bedding for the baby Jesus. The 'Lady' in the name is the Virgin Mary.

How to eat cleavers

Two things have stood out for us in writing about cleavers again. The first is the emergence of bioengineering research into how it can spread so efficiently: new respect for its subtle strengths.

The second thing is just how good cleavers can be to eat, both cooked and in salads, notably in the spring, and just how much we love to drink the cold infusion. It is our 'go to' drink and regular teaching tool in workshops and courses.

Another drink recipe is a cleavers ersatz 'coffee' using the roasted ripe brown seeds.

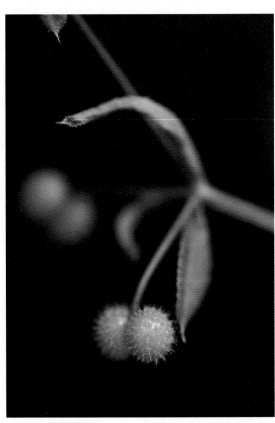

Cleavers **Cold Infusion**

This is a wonderfully refreshing drink that will help keep your lymph clear.

Simply fill a jug with **freshly picked cleavers**. Cut the stems rather than pick them as this will reduce bruising of the plant. Fill the jug with **water**, and leave overnight. The cleavers will stick to itself, so you can just pour out the water you want to drink. More water can be added during the day, but make a fresh batch for the next day.

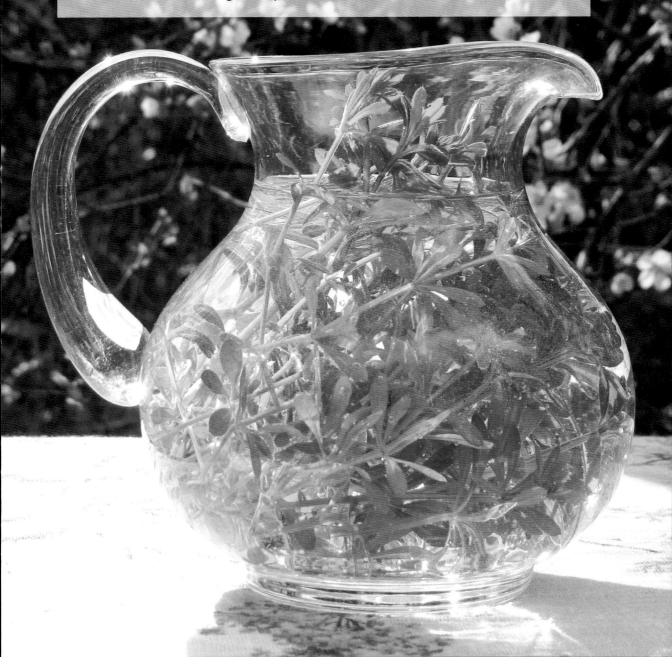

Cleavers **Moussaka**

Harvest a bowlful of cleavers tips. They are at their most succulent just before they flower, when they give a 'meaty' texture. Set aside leftover lentils or cook ½ **cup brown lentils**.

Preheat oven to 175C/350F. Cut **2 red peppers** into quarters. Remove the seeds and place on an oven tray, skin side up. Grill until the skins start to blister and blacken. When they are cool, pull the skins off.

Cut **a small eggplant** into ½cm (¼in) wheels. Lightly oil them and grill until cooked and browned, turning as needed. Blanch **a bowlful of cleavers tips** by cooking briefly in boiling water, for up to a minute, then dip in cold water. Drain.

Start layering ingredients in a small casserole dish. Put the grilled eggplant in the bottom, followed by **300g (1½ cups) cooked lentils** mixed with **1 crushed clove garlic** and **salt to taste**, the peeled red peppers and then the blanched cleavers.

Blend **140g (1 cup) raw cashews** with **250ml (1 cup) water, ¼ teaspoon nutmeg** and **½ teaspoon salt**, and pour over the cleavers. Top with **dry breadcrumbs, sesame seeds** or **hulled hemp seeds**.

Bake for half an hour or until golden on top. Serves 2 to 4.

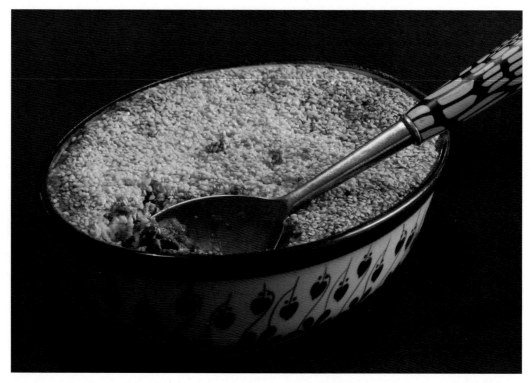

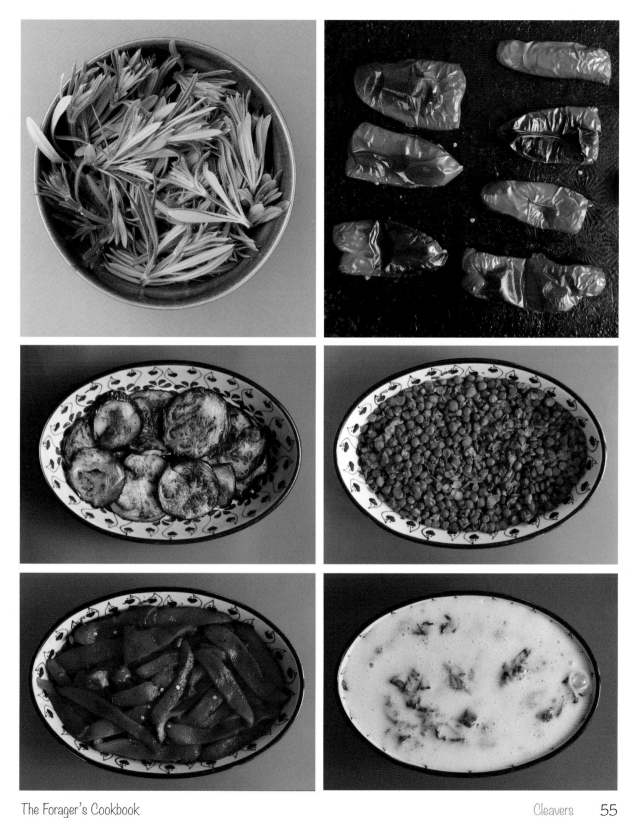

Cleavers Stir Fry

Cleavers tips are at their most succulent just before they flower, but can be picked any time from autumn to late spring. Before you start cooking, prepare your vegetables. They all need to be thinly sliced or cut into bite-sized pieces. These amounts make plenty for two people.

1 red onion, finely sliced
1 large Romano or other red pepper, sliced
a handful or two of green beans
a handful or small bowl of cleavers tips

Heat **a little oil** in a wok. Toasted sesame oil or peanut oil are often used.

Fry the onions and red peppers first as they take longest to cook. Then add the green beans, and lastly the cleavers. Drip in **tamari soy sauce** to taste. The vegetables should be cooked but still have some crunch.

Serve with **noodles** or **rice**.

Alternatives: Cleavers tips can be added to any stir fry. Choose vegetables that will contrast with the green of the cleavers. If you don't have red onions, use regular onion and add some purple cabbage for color. Other greens in season can be used, such as chickweed, wild garlic (ramsons), garlic chives, green onions (scallions) or green garlic tops. Thin strips of carrot are another good addition, as are ginger or galangal. For a more substantial meal, add chunks of tempeh, tofu or some peanuts. The possibilities are boundless: just use what you have.

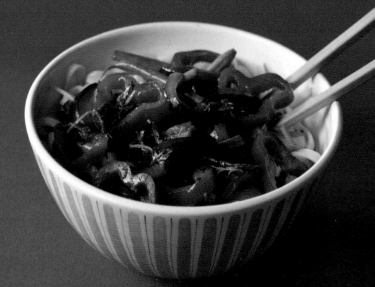

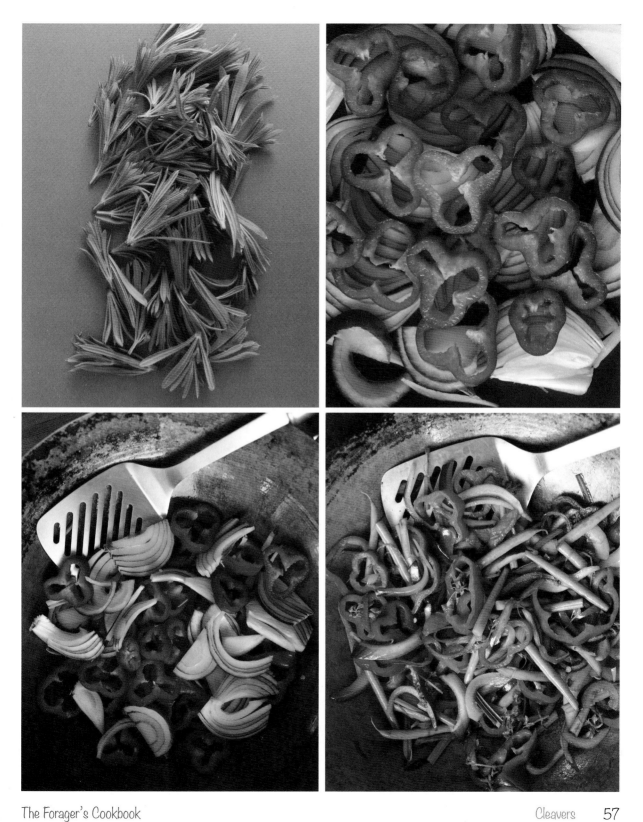

Cresses

The most common weedy cresses in the garden and on road verges are the bittercresses – hairy bittercress (*Cardamine hirsuta*) and wavy bittercress (*C. flexuosa*). Another, found in gardens, in pavements and at field margins, is shepherd's purse (*Capsella bursa-pastoris*). They all have the peppery taste of watercress in milder form.

**Brassicaceae
(formerly Cruciferae)
Cabbage or mustard family**

Annuals.

Edible parts: All above-ground parts when young; later, leaves only. Available from autumn through spring, and all summer in cooler areas.

Distinguishing features: Smallish, low-lying plants that love bare earth, overwintering as a rosette of leaves. Flowers are small, four-petalled in a cruciform shape, white in the bittercresses and shepherd's purse. Bittercress seeds explode out of thin, vertically held dry seedpods. Shepherd's purse has heart-shaped seed pods.

Related edible weeds: Many, including sea rocket, sea kale, wintercresses, yellow cresses, wall rockets and rockets, pepperworts, pennycresses, charlock, white and black mustards, rape, wild turnip, wild cabbage, radish and horseradish, Jack by the hedge, scurvy grasses, honesty and watercress. If happy with your identification, try eating any of these species.

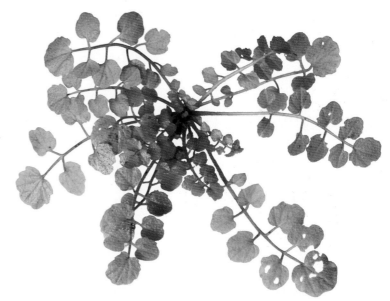

What kind of a weed are bittercresses?

Among numerous edible members of the cabbage or mustard family (see list alongside) we focus on two almost identical common weeds: hairy bittercress (*Cardamine hirsuta*) and wavy bittercress (*C. flexuosa*).

They are abundant in most gardens across the temperate world, self-pollinating, have white flowers with 4 petals, overwinter in bare soil as leaf rosettes, spread explosively, are tasty and best eaten uncooked.

Their English names, unfortunately, are not accurate. Hairy bittercress is only slightly hairy (you need good eyesight or a magnifier to see the small leaf hairs), and the taste is more pungent and peppery than bitter.

The wavy form is often larger than the hairy (to 50cm rather than 30cm, or 20in rather than 12in); the foliage is denser; there are 6 stamens as against 4 in hairy; and, paradoxically, the wavy form has slightly hairy leaves. This being said, you don't need to worry which bittercress you have, as they can both be eaten and taste the same.

Modern genome research shows that the hairy form is the ancestor parent of the wavy form. Hairy bittercress has now become a model species for studying reduced complexity genetics in the cabbage family.

Gardeners dislike the bittercresses because they spring up on bare soil between rows of bedding plants, and as they are frost-hardy, they emerge in winter, before many garden plants get going. Their advantage as pioneers is lost by springtime when rougher and tougher plants take over.

The bittercresses have a special distribution method known as ballistic dispersal. The seedpods are thin and narrow, standing almost vertical on the topmost stems. One website refers to them as toothpick-like.

Differential drying of sections of the seedpod means the pods coil up tightly and, when fully ripe, they explode violently at any touch. No wonder an old name was jumping cress!

Studies by Salisbury (1961) found that the seeds, about 14 to 30 per pod, are projected in all directions in still air to a distance of 90cm (about 3ft); if the wind is gusty they may go further.

There may be several generations of the plants each year, and with good dormancy, give dense ground cover.

The moral is that if you are a grower or gardener, you will strive to avoid your bittercresses going to seed (the adage applies: one year's seeds, seven years of weeds); if you are weed-eater, though, you will encourage it.

The history of bittercress

Their literally explosive methods of spreading meant that the bittercresses were readily able to cross continents. From a probable Eurasian origin they are now known across the temperate world, though the transmission details have been little studied for either prehistoric or historic times.

An interesting modern take on bittercress dispersal is experienced in garden centers. Nurserymen are all too aware how the bare soil of plant containers is a ready seedbed for bittercress to grow, and if allowed to mature the seeds can be projected into adjacent pots. When you buy plants, you may well be receiving free cress!

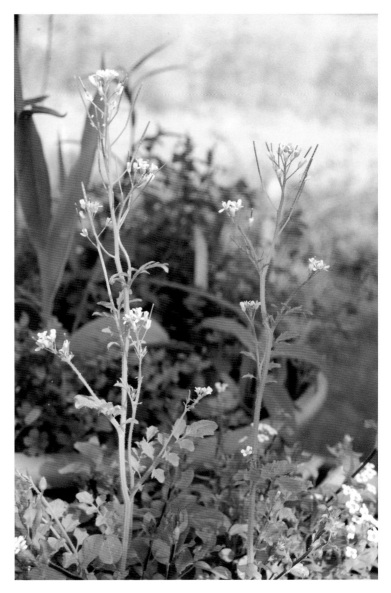

Bittercress flowering in our greenhouse

Bittercress seed is also known to be carried in mulches protecting overwintering plants in gardens as well as nurseries. In a reversal of the usual direction of travel, Asian bittercress (*Cardamine occulta*) and New Zealand bittercress (*C. corymbosa*) are now being recorded as alien incomers in parts of northern England.

One interesting historical note concerns the important role of a bittercress relative, charlock (*Sinapis arvensis*).

The heart-shaped seedpods of shepherd's purse (right) are a clear identifyling feature. Its leaves (below) are very variable in shape.

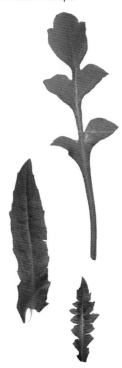

Once a common weed of arable land and some gardens, it has been almost wiped out by chemical herbicides.

Back in Ireland in the 18th century and earlier, however, charlock was a vital survival food, alongside nettle. Known as prashock, it helped fill the 'hungry gap' in May and June before the potato crop was ready.

Before cabbage itself developed as a crop, wild-gathered prashock was sold in the streets of Dublin, and made into a porridge or haggis. One Co. Limerick farmer told the writers Cyril and Kit Ó Céirín (1978) how he still welcomed charlock: *I always save it when weeding the potato field for no cabbage was as sweet.*

Herbal & other uses of bittercress

Some bittercress relatives have been used to combat scurvy – and are still valued for their vitamin C content – such as scurvygrass (*Cochlearia*) species, watercress (*Nasturtium officinale*) and lady's smock or cuckooflower (*Cardamine pratensis*).

Another relative, shepherd's purse (*Capsella bursa-pastoris*), remains an important medicinal herb. Made into a tea, it is used for stopping bleeding, including abnormal menstrual flow. It has a well-established capacity to stimulate uterine contractions, and was resorted to in childbirth. For the same reason it was and should be still avoided in pregnancy itself.

All these bittercress relatives make good peppery eating, though watercress is the only commercially grown and only aquatic species.

How to eat bittercress

We recommend you eat your weedlings! And it's even easier than the mustard and cress you once would have grown on absorbent paper at junior school (in Britain at least). Just keep an eye on bare patches of earth in your garden in winter. The first seedlings to show will often be chickweed, cleavers or hairy bittercress.

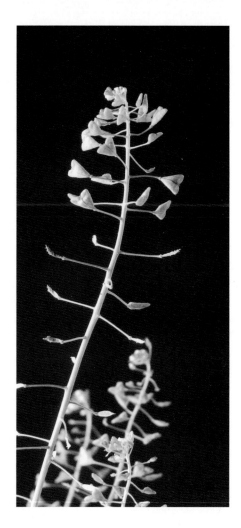

These are nature's microgreens from your own garden, ready to eat (after washing them). Enjoy as a garnish, in salads, sandwiches or a pesto.

For more mature specimens, the best time to harvest the rosette of leaves is before flowering. Cut the stem across, below the rosette and above the tap root. The plant can grow back.

Shepherd's purse is one of the seven herbs used in a Japanese spring soup (see nipplewort chapter).

The pepperiness is destroyed by cooking, so raw is best. Bittercress chemistry has a stimulant effect on digestion, making it an ideal starter.

Cress & Pomegranate **Salad**

Harvest your **bittercress** with a pair of scissors, or if you are pulling up whole rosettes to weed the garden, snip off the individual leaflets once you get it in the house.

Wash the cress to remove any bits of soil that may have stuck to it. Arrange in a bowl with a generous scattering of **pomegranate seeds**. The red and the green provide a vibrant counterpoint, and this simple raw salad is perfect without any dressing.

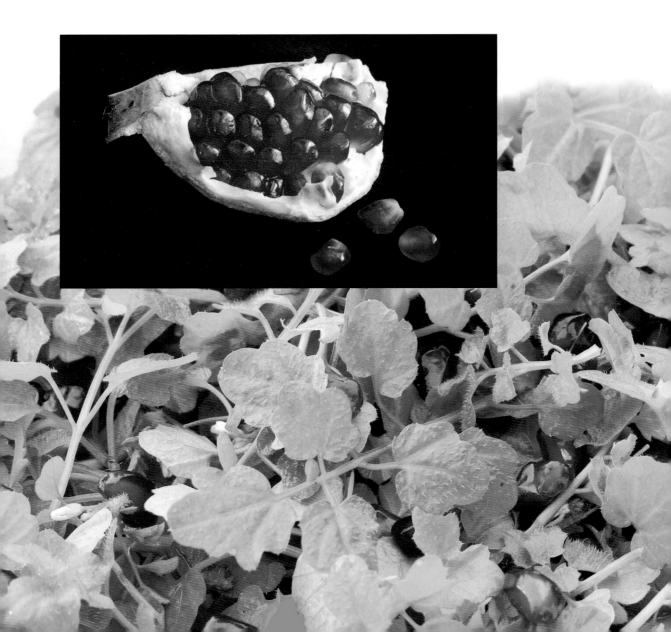

Daisy & Ox-Eye Daisy

Common daisy (*Bellis perennis*) is a weed of lawns and short grass, while the larger ox-eye daisy (*Leucanthemum vulgare*) prefers waysides, road verges and disturbed soil. Both are edible as well as medicinal, and while the leaves of the larger daisy are popular in salads in Italy, they are under-appreciated in Britain and North America. The flowers and petals of both daisies can also be eaten.

**Asteraceae
Daisy family
(formerly Compositae)**

Perennial.

Distinguishing features
Daisy is a small plant, up to 20cm (8in), abounding in long grass and much less in frequently mown lawns. Ox-eye daisy is a taller plant, usually around 50cm (20in), growing in long grass or on disturbed soil.
Daisy's flowerhead opens in sunlight and closes at night (hence the old name 'day's eye'), whereas the larger ox-eye flowers stay open day and night.

Daisy begins to flower in early spring, ox-eye in late spring and early summer.

Both have rosettes of succulent green leaves all year.

*Wel by reason men it call maie
The daisie or els the eye of the daie.*
– Chaucer (c1386)

What kind of weeds are daisies?

Children of all ages – and poets led by Chaucer – love daisies, as flowers of carefree summers when it was time to make daisy chains or garlands.

Gardeners and farmers, though, have been less enthusiastic in welcoming the white and gold flowerheads of common (or field or English) daisy and its larger relative, the ox-eye daisy.

Both plants had their origin in Europe and across Asia, but it is outside these native areas that they were introduced, often as garden species, and escaped to become invasive weeds, across North America, in Australasia and in parts of Africa and South America.

In each case these plants have dense and overlapping basal leaf rosettes, which effectively restrict nutrients and light from reaching competing plants, and sustain daisy colonies. Neither plant develops 'parachutes' to fly the seeds away from the parent plant, so the many seeds fall close by and swell the local population.

There is a lovely custom in parts of Britain that spring arrives when your foot can cover seven, nine or sometimes twelve daisy flowers (it varies in different areas). Given how close the neighboring plants usually are, this reassuringly means that spring is inevitable.

Daisy has a clever method for surviving in lawns: it keeps its basal leaves snug to the earth and below the level of garden mowers' blades. Another trick is quick flowering and the fact that each flower emerges out of a stem that can be of variable height.

You can find daisies in well-mown lawns flowering while hugging the ground, but when there is no mowing the flower stem will be much taller.

Ox-eye adopts a different strategy, in growing tall (up to a meter or 3.3ft), and achieving maximum density of flowering blooms. A pasture or meadow in a bright summer might be overwhelmingly full of millions of the plants: a delight for the walker but a disaster for the farmer.

A mature ox-eye plant can produce up to 26,000 seeds a year. It spreads both by seeds and by rhizomes, which can replicate even from a small piece.

An intriguing Anglo-French research project into meadow flowers led by Damien Hicks (2016) found that ox-eye plants produced more pollen per flowerhead than any other species – no wonder ox-eye-full fields are insect-loud in midsummer.

Some gardeners even welcome an outbreak of daisies in the lawn, as such a sudden appearance can be an indication of a soil deficient in lime.

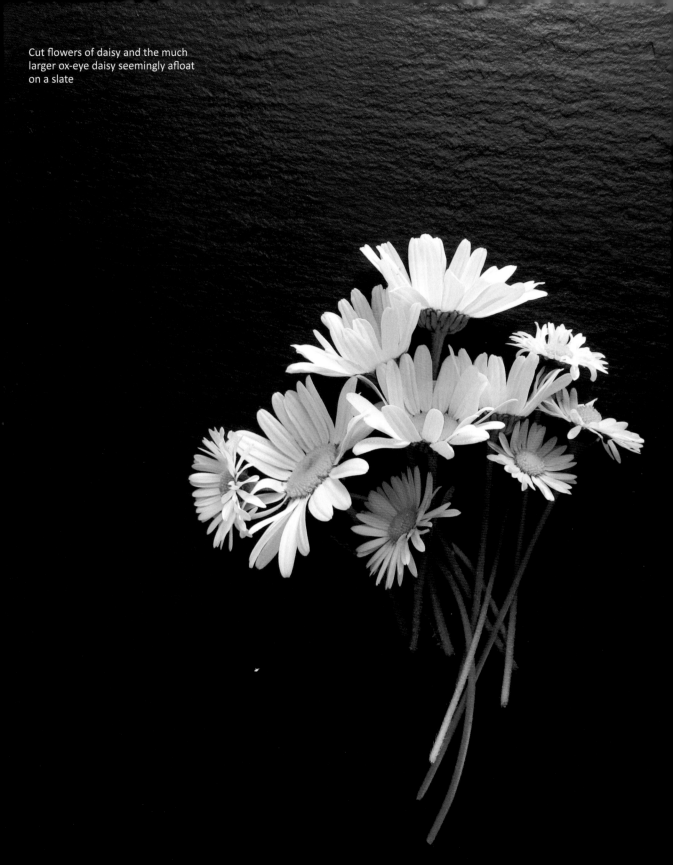

Cut flowers of daisy and the much larger ox-eye daisy seemingly afloat on a slate

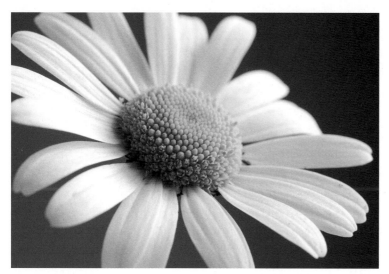

Ox-eye daisy flower, showing the individual disc florets and their spiral arrangement

[Ox-eye is] *a terrific and unusual-tasting salad plant.*

– Rensten (2016)

Daisies are rich in calcium and, as they die and decompose, their remains enrich the soil. Allowing a cycle of daisies to rebalance an over-acid soil may be a mark of wise husbandry.

The history of daisy and ox-eye daisy

The archaeological record says little on the presence of either species in prehistory, though it is likely they flourished where there were meadows and grazed pastures.

In ancient Rome the first-century AD naturalist Pliny writes of daisy, but

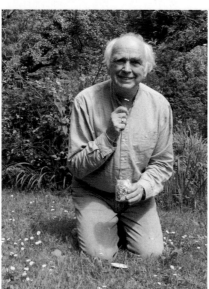

Right: Matthew, happily harvesting daisy for tea. Opposite: even stately homes have daisies in the lawn

only to say briefly it is a pretty, white meadow plant. He adds, rather too cryptically: *It is held that an application of it is more efficacious* [ie herbally] *if Artemisia is added.*

Daisy was a Roman wound-cure herb, with bandages soaked in daisy tea deployed to treat cuts, bruises and flesh wounds from the battlefield.

We have used it as an ointment for bruises and cysts ourselves, and have found that mugwort (our most common *Artemisia*, and included in this book) enhances the already strong healing action of daisy.

It's not clear whether Pliny is referring to military or civilian uses. In any case, daisy was well known to him, and he calls it *Bellis*, a name that has stuck. And no wonder – it means 'beautiful'.

There is a minority view, espoused by the herbalist W.T. Fernie (1897), among others, that daisy is *Bellis* because the word also means 'war', since daisy was used as a healing herb in that context, much like yarrow (named *Achillea* after the famed general Achilles).

It is somehow hard, though, to imagine Linnaeus, the great classifier of plants, settling his name of *Bellis perennis* on daisy, in 1753, as meaning 'perpetual war' rather than 'beautiful forever'.

Daisy was a plant of the moon in classical times, dedicated to Artemis (Greece) and Diana (Rome). Ox-eye is still sometimes called moon daisy.

As Christianity replaced the old gods and goddesses, so plants were renamed too. By medieval times, our two plants had new patrons: daisy had become herb Margaret and ox-eye was maudlinewort.

Herb Margaret name-checked Margaret of Cortona, a 13th-century Franciscan saint from Italy, patron of homeless people and outsiders (possibly weeds too?). She was prayed to for recovery from uterine complaints, and daisy tea was used for that purpose.

Ox-eye's name maudlinewort referred to Mary Magdalene; the plant was also known as great marguerite, midsummer daisy and St John's flower (St John's day is 24 June), gypsies' daisy, dog daisy and false sunflower.

Another identity it once had was Buphthalmum, but this name (as *Buphthalmum salicifolium*) now describes yellow ox-eye daisy, a European native and garden flower.

The first written example of 'daisy' in English is recorded by the *OED* as around the year 1000, in a Saxon leechbook (medical recipes). 'Ox-eye', by contrast, first appears around 1400.

Our two plant names, however, had become overly long and descriptive in both English and Latin by the time of the last great herbal in English, John Parkinson's *Theatrum Botanicum* (1640).

He described 12 types of daisy, with daisy itself being the Lesser white wild Daisie (*Bellis minor sylvestris simplex*) and ox-eye the Great white wild Daisie (*Bellis major vulgaris sive sylvestris*). It was time for Linnaeus to intervene.

Modern renaming, though, has been unkind to ox-eye: once the euphonious *Chrysanthemum leucanthemum* (gold flower, white flower) of Linnaeus, it is now *Leucanthemum vulgare* (common white flower).

Herbal & other uses of daisy and ox-eye daisy

The two daisies are often considered equivalent by herbalists; in the words of Henry Lyte (1578), *there are two kinds of Daysies, the great and small.*

There is a difference in intensity, perhaps. Parkinson (1640) points out that *the small daisy is held to be more astringent and binding than any other* [of the daisies]. This astringency comes through in the taste of the leaves, daisy being less palatable as summer goes on.

We have noted already that daisy, and by extension ox-eye, were wound herbs and used for uterine issues. They were given as a tea, ointment or poultice.

It is useful information that if you have daisy and yarrow in your garden (and many of us do), you have excellent healing potential at hand for wounds, bleeding and shock.

Daisy tea has an old folk reputation for relieving chronic coughs and bronchial catarrhs. It has a high level of vitamin C – about the same as lemons – and is a depurative, ie it makes you sweat.

In some respiratory conditions, such as pleurisy, drinking hot daisy tea, while in bed, swathed in blankets, may help in breaking the fever.

For blocked nasal passages the herbalist Juliette de Baïracli Levy (1974) recommends wilting daisy leaves, allowing them to cool, rolling them into balls and pushing them up the nose.

She says, keep them there as long as can be tolerated. Chewing the fresh leaves can help soothe mouth ulcers.

Ox-eye is known as an antispasmodic, being used to soothe whooping cough

How daisy won a queen's heart

An old Greek story explains how daisy won the heart of Rose, the queen of the flowers.

Rose had a birthday party and all the flowers were invited. One little flower was left behind, however. It was shy because of its modest appearance and whispered its congratulations from far away.

But the wind carried the flower's words to the queen, who assured daisy that there was no need to be ashamed: its dress was spotlessly white and it had a heart of gold.

This made the little flower blush, and ever since that day the tips of its ray florets have been tinged with pink.

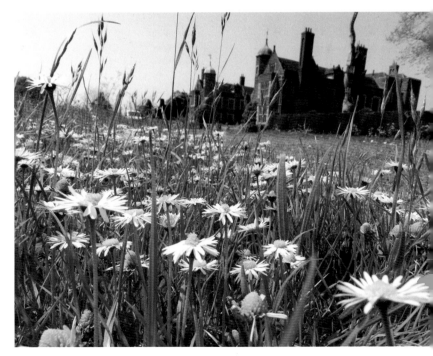

or asthma; it is more specific than daisy for night sweats.

As well as bruises (another old name is bruisewort), daisy tea can be drunk and, once cool, applied externally as a poultice or ointment for stiff neck and lumbago, various aches or stiffness.

Daisy is a wonderful pain reliever, the 'poor man's arnica'. Arnica (*Arnica montana*) is well known in self-help pain management, but the plant is endangered, expensive and has toxicity issues. Daisy is preferable in every way.

Daisy tea can be used in a spray bottle as an insect repellant.

Modern research is steadily confirming daisy's time-honored benefits, including in wound-healing, and potential as an antioxidant, antimicrobial and antitumor aid, including for human digestive tract carcinoma (see our *Wayside Medicine*).

Daisy has a benign reputation, and is safe for children, a fact reflected in yet another old name, bairnwort.

But take note that as an introduced alien plant in the American West and Australia ox-eye might cause contact dermatitis in sensitive skins. The hotter drier conditions in these regions may intensify the chemistry of the plant.

Daisy itself can arouse allergic reactions to its pollen, but this is more likely in the related garden aster flower or chamomile.

Daisy is best avoided in pregnancy.

How to eat daisy and ox-eye daisy

A search in the herbal and cookery literature suggests that common daisy has never been a go-to wild food, even in times of famine. The taste is a little too soapy and bitter for most people, as compared with the more popular use of the tender leaves of ox-eye daisy.

The leaves are available almost year round, while the flowers have a much shorter season. Commonly daisy flowers in the spring, and ox-eye flowers for about a month at mid-summer, though both produce the odd flower out of season.

For **soups**, use the youngest leaves of either plant where tenderness has not been supplanted by bitterness.

The French garden writer Jean Palaiseul (1973) likes daisy leaves as a green vegetable and stewed with meat, *thus pleasing the palate and loosening the bowels at the same time.*

In **salads** both daisy and ox-eye are less bitter than dandelion leaves and can serve to modify its taste. The bright white of the flower petals is a visual delight as a salad garnish.

The urban forager John Rensten (2016) says leaves of lime tree and ox-eye form his favorite spring salad, with a dash of rosehip vinegar.

The flower buds of both plants can be **pickled** or put fresh in a **sandwich** or **salad**, in the same manner as capers.

Adding strong flavors to a daisy or ox-eye dish is a good strategy to balance the taste, as we do in our raita recipe (p68).

The young leaves [of daisy] are eaten raw or cooked, they have a reasonable mild flavor but are often a bit tough and are far from my favorite leaf. ... The flower buds and petals can also be eaten in salads, they are very decorative but look much nicer than they taste.
– Fern (2000)

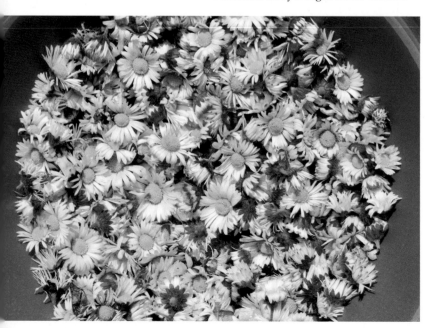

Daisy Tea

Daisy tea is calming like chamomile tea, a relative. The taste is mild and pleasant.

Pick **a handful of daisy flowers** and put them in a teapot. Pour **boiling water** over them, put the lid on the teapot, and leave to brew for 5 to 10 minutes.

Strain and enjoy.

Alternatives: Dried daisy flowers can also be used. Also nice with fennel seed or mint.

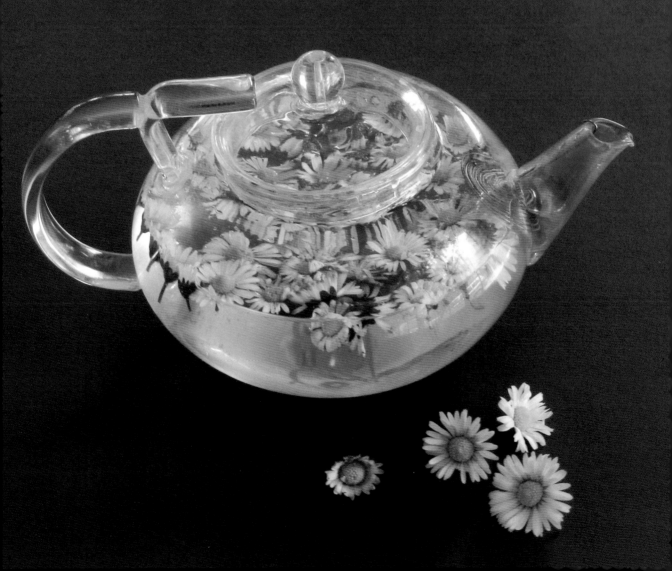

Daisy **Raita**

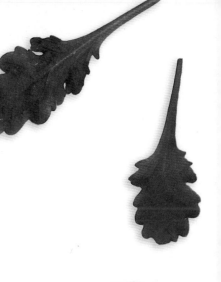

This is a lovely cooling accompaniment to serve with hot spicy food or as part of a mezze.

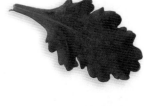

Mix together:
235g (1 cup) thick coconut yogurt
8g (¼ cup) finely chopped ox-eye daisy leaves & daisy leaves
1 clove garlic, crushed
salt and pepper to taste

Serve at room temperature for the best flavor.

Alternatives: Try adding a little bit of finely chopped ground ivy leaves. Sorrel is also really tasty in a raita.

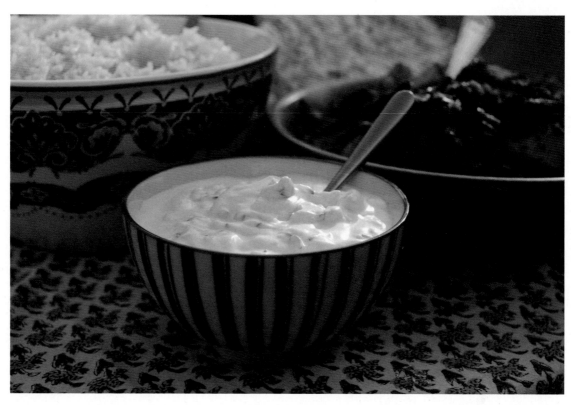

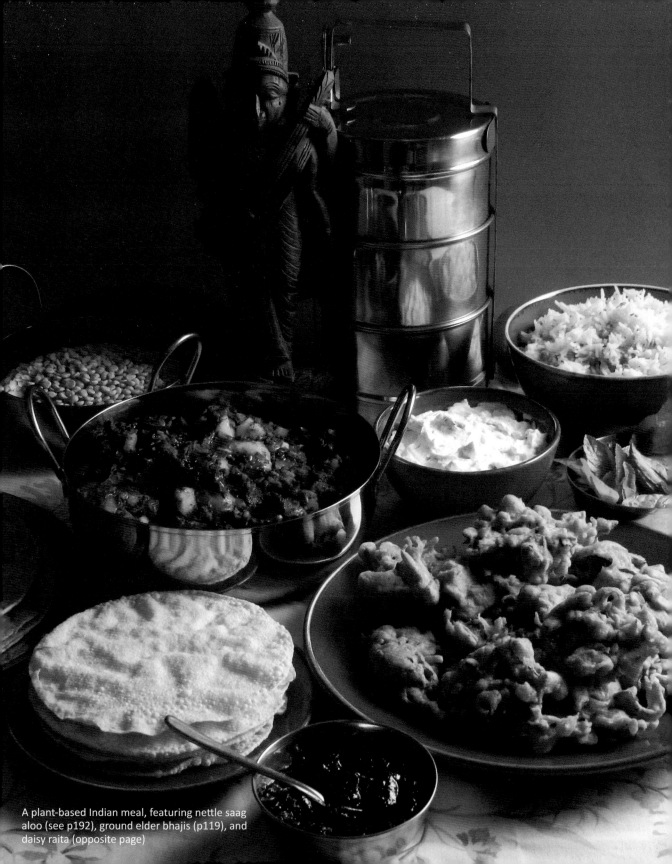

A plant-based Indian meal, featuring nettle saag aloo (see p192), ground elder bhajis (p119), and daisy raita (opposite page)

Dandelion

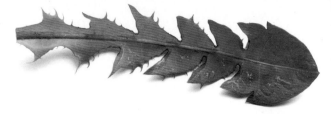

Named for the lion, dandelion (*Taraxacum officinale* agg.) is a king of bitters, veritable herbal royalty. A cosmopolitan presence in temperate latitudes, it is so well known that it becomes invisible, unless as a troublesome garden weed. We want to help reclaim it as a wonderful wild food, and we feature both savory and sweet offerings, as well as a sparkling drink.

Asteraceae (formerly Compositae) Daisy family

Perennial.

Edible parts: Whole plant, including roots. Leaves are best in spring, flowers are most abundant in spring, and root best dug in autumn.

Distinguishing features: Leaves emerge from the top of the taproot to form a basal rosette; jagged lobes inspired the 'teeth of the lion' name, although some leaves are entire (unindented); sunburst yellow flower; flower closes at night; stems pale green, hairless or gently fuzzy, hollow with bitter white latex; long brown tap root; 'clock' of fruit with individual parachutes, leaving a domed 'monk's head' once dispersed.

Edible relatives: Chicory, the hawkbits, burdock, spear thistle, the sowthistles, daisy and ox-eye daisy, nipplewort, mugwort, yarrow. Several of these feature in this book.

What kind of a weed is dandelion?

Dandelion (*Taraxacum officinale* agg.) is an ultimate cosmopolitan weed, sun-spreading its way across the temperate north and south. Native to Eurasia and probably North America, it has spread prodigiously to become perhaps the most recognizable 'worldwide weed'.

We've seen it throughout our travels, and like to photograph the dandelions of every new place we visit. The image opposite was taken in the Italian Alps.

We want to highlight nine elements of weedness in dandelion's success as a wild plant/weed:

1. Its long tap root is often a meter (3.3ft) deep, and more in some North American dandelions. It's hard work pulling it out or digging it up. The French author Pierre Morency (1992) rightly says dandelion has 'one of the firmest grips on life' of any plant.

Its deep root system not only fixes dandelion in the earth but opens up a channel for minerals drawn up from below; these minerals benefit us when we eat any of the plant.

2. Dandelion's compact and low-to-the-ground rosette of basal leaves shades out competing plants, and its roots produce chemicals that inhibit germination in ryegrass and other meadow plants (this is known as an allelopathic effect).

3. Another protection is dandelion's bitterness (see below).

4. The roots can regenerate from the least scrap left behind in the soil. So zealous gardeners who behead their dandelions in the lawn by mowing will not be rid of them.

5. Dandelion does not need to be fertilized and can reproduce directly from the ovule (that is, no male assistance is needed). In this process, called apomixis, offspring are clones of the parent, while random mutations in the cells can still occur.

6. Beneficial survival traits are selectively retained from the mutations, leading to a proliferation of subtly different dandelion microspecies. One count (Stace 2010) found 234 microspecies in Britain alone.

Officially *Taraxacum officinale* is called an 'aggregate' (agg.). Botanists may spend an anguished (or fulfilled) lifetime 'splitting' the microspecies, but as our focus is on eating we will be 'lumpers' and treat *T. officinale* collectively as one food source.

7. Dandelions produce plentiful pollen and nectar, as an important source of nutrition for early spring insects. Microspecies in some places do reproduce sexually (or else why would pollen and nectar still be needed at all?) in another survival strategy.

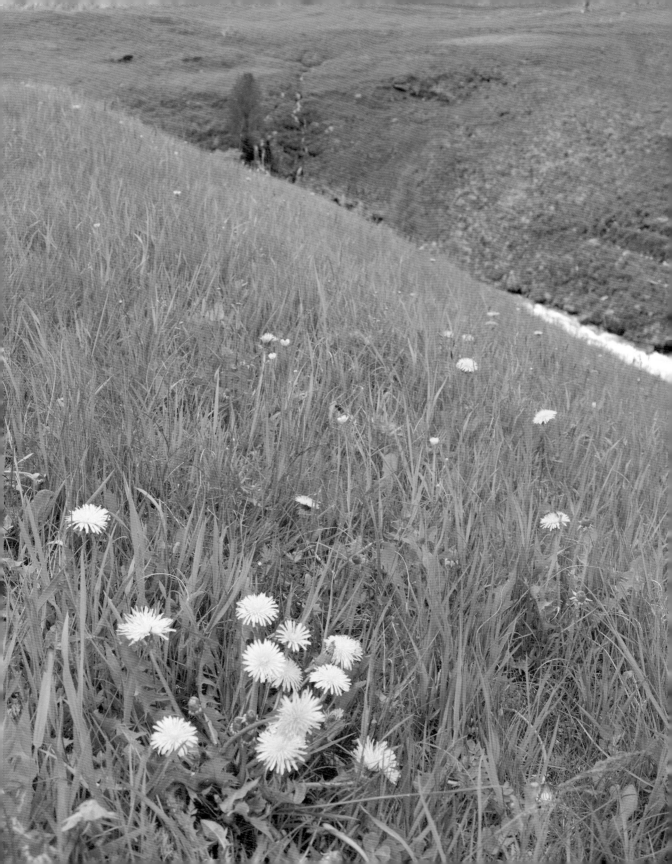

8. Then the seeds can fly. We all know the dandelion 'clock' game of blowing the parachutes of fruits away, making a wish as we do so.

One dandelion flowerhead is actually a collection of up to 200 separate individual flowers, each producing its own fruit (what we think of as the seed). These units make a composite, giving rise to the old family name Compositae.

Each unit develops its own bristly parachute (pappus) to be carried on the wind a few meters or kilometers away from the parent.

With several flower stalks per plant and a meadow full of dandelions, there can be millions of parachutes, enabling a massive potential distribution.

Scientists in Edinburgh recently found that the parachutes have a unique form of flight not known before in nature (Cummins 2018).

The bristles of the pappus are so spaced that an air bubble forms, known as the separated vortex ring, and this is stabilized as air flows through it. The bubble delays the descent of the seed to the ground, in a mechanism the researchers say is four times more efficient than the most advanced human parachute design.

9. Add to all this that dandelion is perennial, and you have huge survival and distribution power.

The history of dandelion

Proto-dandelions have been dated to about 30 million years ago, and fossil fruit of *Taraxacum tanaiticum* from the Pliocene (between 5 and 2.5 million years ago) has been found in Russia.

There are abundant survivals of the fruit of *T. officinale* in interglacial and glacial periods in Britain over the last million years. Sir Harry Godwin, historian of the British flora (1956), talks of 'a pattern of persistence' through to the present.

Dandelion was known in ancient Egypt, classical Greece and Rome, as well as imperial China and Japan, both as food and medicine.

Perhaps surprisingly, the written record really begins in another culture, the Persian empire of around a thousand years ago. The physician al-Razi, known in the West as Rhazes (AD 854–925), wrote of *tarashaquq*, a plant like chicory. This could be where the name *taraxacum* originates.

Another Persian scientist who elaborated on dandelion was Ibn Sina (in the West, Avicenna) (AD 980–1037). When his medical encyclopedia was translated into Latin in 1170 the plant was identified as *tarasacon*.

An old English name for dandelion is Persian bitter herb, which may reflect a hazy line of transmitted knowledge about its medicinal value.

In North America questions remain whether dandelion has a native origin, was transported across the land-bridge in Alaska (Beringia) in the last Ice Age or was introduced by European immigrants, as a useful medicinal or accidentally in clothes or fodder.

It could also have flown in on the jet stream. In any event, the plant was soon incorporated into Cree, Apache and Mohican medicine, among others.

When Linnaeus (1707–78) systematized the known natural world, he classified dandelion as *Leontedon taraxacum*. This name was changed later to *Taraxacum officinale*, the form now used; the Leontedons were reclassified as the hawkbits, which are close dandelion relatives and also edible.

'Dandelion', the English form of the French 'dent de lion', is another version of Leontedon. Most commentators suggest this comes from the jagged appearance of some of the basal leaves, which reminded people of the animal's teeth. We edge closer to American herbal writer Maida Silverman (1997), who notes that when calling dandelion to mind we think first of the sun-like flower and not the leaves. The English poet Robert Bridges had no doubts: in his paean to wild flowers, 'The Idle Flowers' (1912), we find *shock-headed Dandelion / that drank the fire of the sun*.

Historically dandelion has been a survival food (see the Cleghorn quote opposite) and is still a wild-gathered plant marketed as an edible green leaf in spring and summer, especially in mainland Europe.

It is also a commercial crop in modern-day Eastern Europe, China and pockets of East Coast North America.

Dandelion has further potential as an alternative to rubber trees in producing rubber from the latex. The species used is *Taraxacum kok-saghyz* (known, mercifully, as TKS), which has exceptional quantities of latex, and new cultivars may further increase the level of output.

This intriguing new role for dandelion has been researched in Russia and the US, and money has been thrown at it since at least the First World War, with trials resuming whenever Southeast Asian supplies of *Hevea braziliensis*, the rubber tree, are threatened by war, disease or price rises.

Rubber-making is a tantalizing prospect for a new era in dandelion's history. It currently remains expensive to harvest for this purpose, but useful by-products might well include biomass and inulin.

Herbal & other uses of dandelion

Written records and oral traditions have long linked dandelion's value as food and medicine.

If asked to summarize its medicinal effect in one word, 'clearing' might be ours. Imagine a Mediterranean rural meal including boiled dandelion greens. The bitterness of the leaves stimulates the taste buds and digestive fire, and lends savor to the appetite.

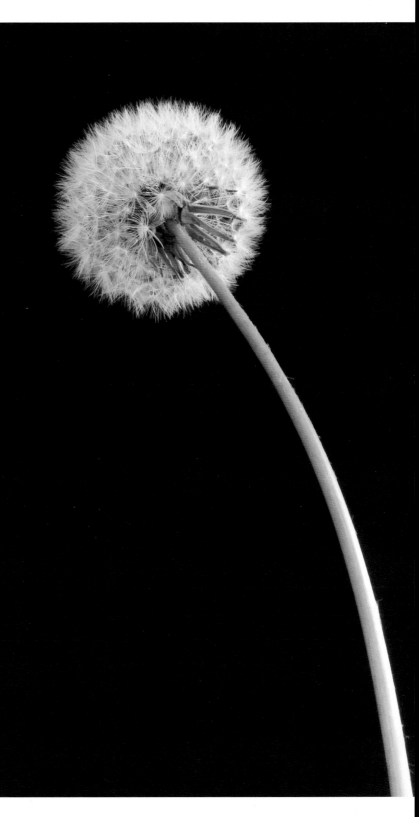

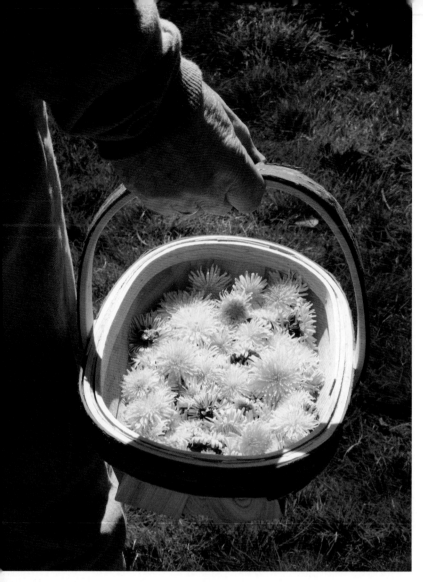

Its bitterness helps make dandelion a liver herb par excellence, and the leaf is still approved (*officinale* in the name means 'official') as a choloretic, or bile enhancer, in the *British Herbal Pharmacopoeia* (1996); the root is also 'official' in the same listing as an hepatic or general liver herb.

In North America dandelion was approved in the *US Pharmacopoeia* from 1830 to 1920; it is under review for readmission.

What is good for the liver is often good for the skin, and dandelion can be taken to ease skin eruptions, rashes and eczema.

Dandelion root contains a high measure of inulin, a recognized supplement in helping reduce vascular fat and hence promoting weight loss.

Then there is dandelion's well-known diuretic effect. It gave the old name piss-a-bed in England and the still-current French piss-en-lit, and similar terms in most European languages.

Whenever you take dandelion, especially as a tea, be prepared to have your kidneys 'cleared by urine', as older herbals put it, and make those regular trips to the toilet. Dandelion flushes out both water and waste products.

Dandelion leaves contain potassium in large quantities (some 4.5%). Unlike diuretic drugs, which leach out the body's potassium, dandelion adds to the body's reservoir of this important element even as it increases urine flow.

If you have water retention, or edema, dandelion could be a remedy an herbalist recommends.

Another old term used for dandelion, 'deobstruent', highlights this cleansing or, in larger quantities, purging element of dandelion's action. But this is not mere elimination.

Dandelion's long tap root brings up many minerals and chemical elements that suffuse the above-ground parts of the plant. For example, the leaves contain high levels of vitamin C, attested by an old dandelion reputation to treat scurvy.

It is one of our most beautiful native plants, and, if not so common, would doubtless be highly valued, but is one of the most troublesome weeds in the field and garden.
– Pierpoint Johnson (1862)

In the stomach the bitterness helps release digestive juices, which work through the organs to the liver, kidneys and bowel.

The bitterness is a part of dandelion's protective allelopathic effect, shared by many Asteraceae. In dandelion and chicory, the bitter-tasting latex effectively deters other plants, insects, grazing animals and helminths.

Dandelion's bitterness peaks late in the day, so if gathering the flowers for our dandelion nuggets recipe (see p78), do so before midday if you want them to be readily palatable.

Vitamin K is present in such quantity in dandelion that taking even a modest amount of the plant in some form meets the body's daily needs several times over. Vitamin K is significant in blood clotting, for protein metabolism and healthy bones and teeth.

Dandelion contains nearly all the other vitamins and most necessary minerals, in bioavailable form, which contributes to its status as a weed superfood and herbal royalty. The overall effect was described in older books as 'cleansing the blood'.

It also has an important contribution to the hormonal system, including in the pancreas, so participating in regulating blood sugar and insulin, and a potential role in type 2 diabetes control. At the same time, people with diabetes should be cautious about taking dandelion if their blood sugar balance could be disturbed.

The *Review of Diabetic Studies* in 2016 published a paper by Wirngo et al., which suggested that dandelion offers a compelling profile of bioactive components with potential anti-diabetic properties. The paper notes that human trials, though, are lacking.

Dandelion is non-toxic, safe and with few side effects, though it may cause allergic reactions in those sensitive to other daisy family plants.

How to eat dandelion

All parts of dandelion are edible, except perhaps the seed parachutes.

The flowers are most abundant for a couple of weeks in spring, but there will be a few around for most of the year, especially if the dandelions have been mowed.

The leaves can be picked much of the year but are at their best in spring, especially for salads. In summer, look for dandelions growing in cool shady locations, as they will be more succulent and less bitter than those growing in full sun and dry soil.

If the bitterness of dandelion greens worries you, here is help from Dr John Kallas. In a web essay in 2003 he offered four techniques for increasing dandelion's palatability.

First is **diluting**: mix it with milder greens like chickweed; next, **masking**: adding fats reduces any harshness and enhances flavor; third is **distracting**: add sugar, vinegar or other strong flavoring; then **blanching**, boiling the greens for a few minutes reduces bitterness.

The latter is a cooking method traditionally adopted in Mediterranean countries where a whole rosette of leaves is often cut with the top part of the root attached, then boiled, sometimes soaking first and changing the water several times. Once cooked, the greens are served with olive oil and lemon juice.

We can suggest two more techniques: cover your growing dandelions with a large flower pot to **exclude light** and blanch them; and **lacto-ferment** your dandelions, as in a sauerkraut.

Of course, you can always grin and bear it, thinking of the beneficial vitamins, fiber and minerals that the bitter leaves are bringing you. And some people really enjoy bitter flavors – we are all different.

Dandelion root coffee is a traditional health drink, again benefiting the liver, and is commercially available. It is very similar to chicory root coffee. But if you are a gardener and wanting to dig up some of your dandelions, you can make your own. Roots are best harvested in the autumn and winter, but can be dug at any time you need them. Wash and chop them, then roast in the oven on a baking tray at a low temperature until dry.

By making our food rich with the wisdom of the dandelion, the intrinsic medicinal values are integrated into our lifestyles as a bonus.
– Blair (2014)

A shot of pure Dandelion juice is somewhat reminiscent of a shot of espresso, the bitterness awakening, stimulating, moving and penetrating: a wake-up call to all the cells in the body.
– Hughes (2016)

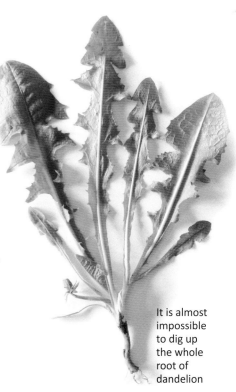

It is almost impossible to dig up the whole root of dandelion

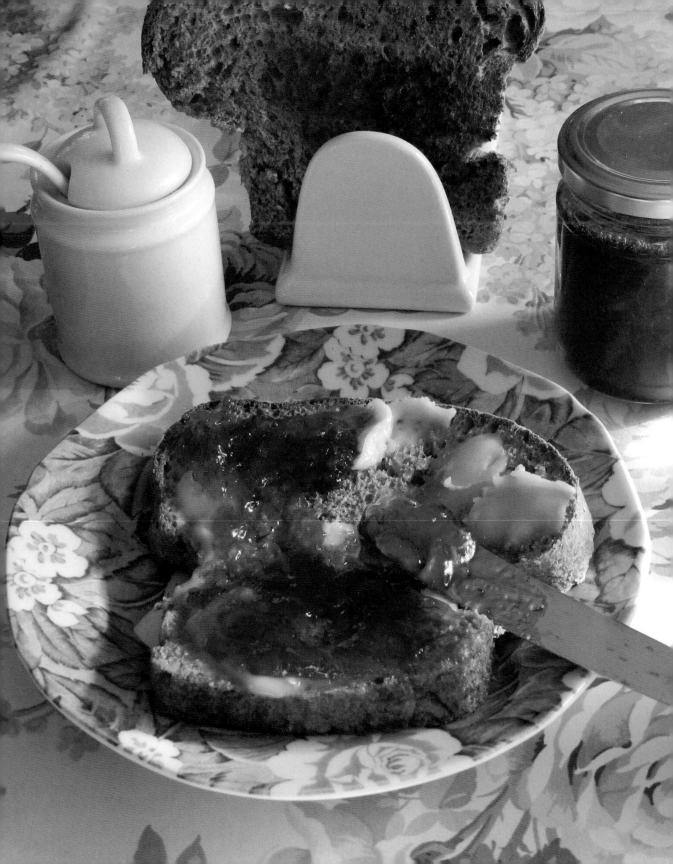

Dandelion Flower **Jam**

This jam is based on a traditional French recipe, called *crémaillotte* (also spelled *cramaillote/ cramaillotte*, or known as *confiture de pissenlits*). You can filter out the flower petals for a clear jam, which is called *miel de pissenlit* (dandelion honey), or leave them in as we do in this recipe, which is more like a marmalade. Some recipes include apple, but we have used jam sugar (sugar with added pectin). Makes about 800ml (1½ pints).

Remove the petals from **a colander full of dandelion flowers**. You can either pull them off the base of the flower, or use a knife to cut them. Put the petals in a saucepan with **500ml (17fl oz) water** and simmer for 10 minutes, then add **the juice of 2 medium lemons** and **600g (21oz) jam sugar** (or mix ordinary sugar with 2 teaspoons pectin powder).

Bring rapidly to a rolling boil, and continue until the setting point is reached (105C/220F). If you don't have a cooking thermometer, test a drop of the jam on a cold saucer after about 5 minutes of rapid boiling. If it gels, the jam is ready. If it doesn't, continue boiling and test again every few minutes until the jam sets on the cold saucer.

When it is ready, add the **finely grated zest of the 2 lemons.** Let it sit for about 10 minutes before pouring into heated jam jars, filling each to the top. This is to allow it to thicken slightly so the petals don't all float to the top. Once set, put the lids on and add a label. Will keep for six months to a year, but refrigerate once opened.

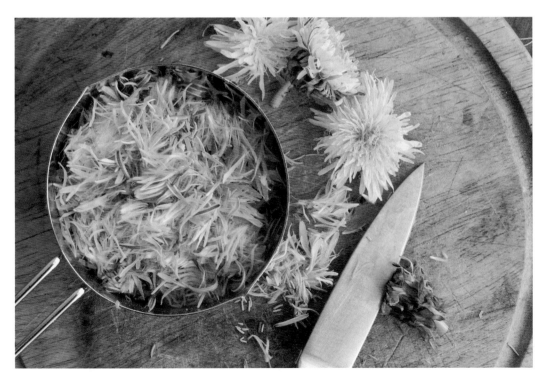

Dandelion Flower **Nuggets**

Every year we look forward to the two or three weeks in April when dandelion flowers are abundant enough to have them for lunch. We say for lunch because they become bitter if picked in the evening – if you like bitter tastes, that's not a problem – but they are tastier if gathered on a warm sunny morning.

Pick enough **dandelion flowers** to allow about a dozen per person, depending what else you are serving with them. Wash them in water, then shake off the excess and roll the flowers while they are still wet in a bowl of **flour or gram flour** (or chickpea/garbanzo flour). Fry in **a little oil** until they are browned on each side. **Salt to taste.**

Serve hot, with a salad and whatever else you like. The taste is more breaded mushroom than dandelion, and they are remarkably good.

Alternatives: Add some chopped herbs to your flour mixture, and cook the flowers with garlic. If you use gram flour, they will be gluten-free.

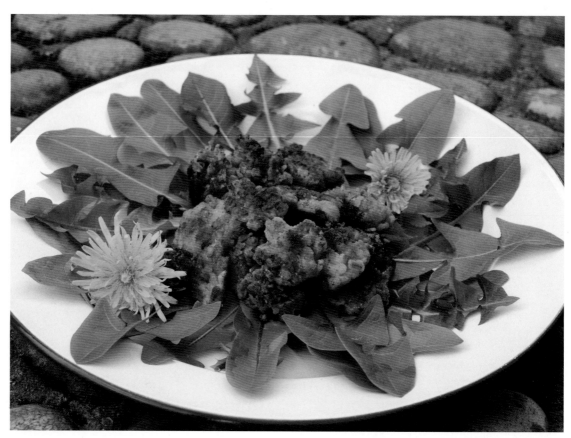

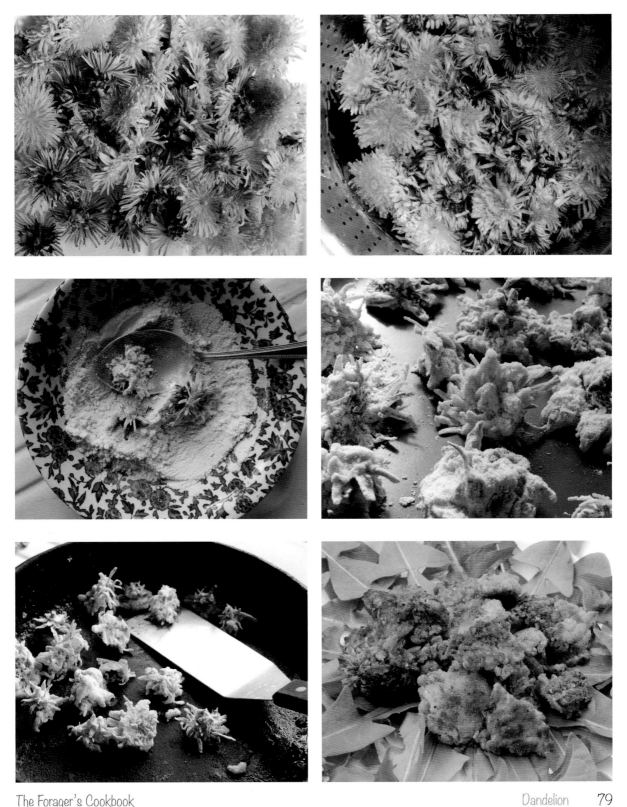

Dandelion Greens & **Noodles**

The combination of fresh spring greens with garlic, ginger and toasted sesame oil is delicious, and the flavors balance the potential bitterness of the herbs. You can use all dandelion leaves or a selection of greens. Add fresh mushrooms or dried honey mushroom – just soak them in hot water for a few minutes.

Allow these amounts per person, so double the amounts if you are cooking for two.

2 good handfuls of dandelions and other spring greens (such as chicory and nipplewort).
Coarsely chop the greens and boil in water for 2 or 3 minutes. The nipplewort won't need long, so add it towards the end. Drain and rinse with **cold water**, then squeeze dry.

Cook **100g (3½ oz) sen lek (brown rice noodles)** or other noodles of choice according to the package directions.

Put **a couple of teaspoons of oil** in a wok or pan.
Add the chopped cooked greens and:
    1 clove garlic, finely grated or minced
    2cm (1in) piece of fresh ginger, finely grated
    a couple of mushrooms, finely sliced

Cook until the mushrooms are done, then add the cooked noodles and toss with **soy sauce** and **a few teaspoons of toasted sesame oil** to taste and serve sprinkled with **black sesame seed**.

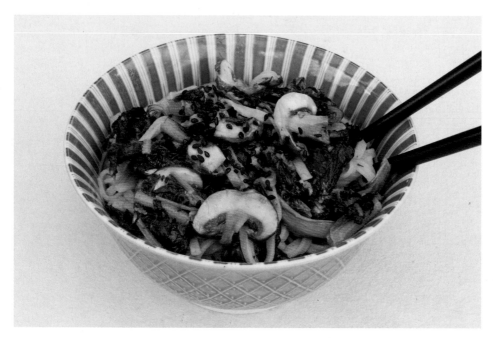

Dandelion Flower **Syrup**

We use this recipe with the dandelion cake on the next page, but this syrup is also delicious on pancakes and waffles, ice cream or with fruit salad.

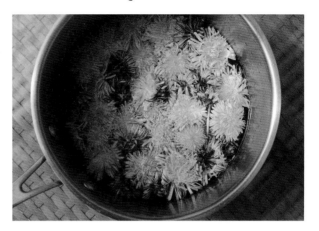

Put **dandelion flowers** in a saucepan with **water** to cover. Add some **sliced lemon** and **orange** (especially delicious with blood orange).

Bring to the boil and simmer about 10 minutes, then set aside to cool – ideally leave it overnight.

Strain the liquid into a measuring jug or cups to see how much you have, then add an equal amount of **light demerara or other sugar**.

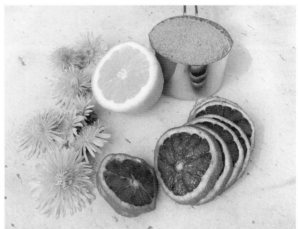

Put liquid back in your saucepan and bring to the boil, stirring until the sugar has all dissolved.

Cool slightly, then pour into heated glass bottles. The syrup can be used straight away or kept until winter, when it will bring sunshine to the darkest of days.

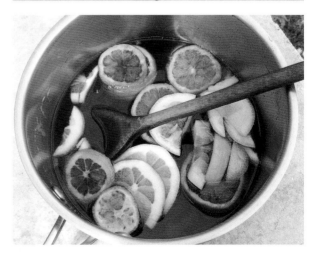

Dandelion Flower Cake

This gluten-free cake makes good use of the spring abundance of dandelion flowers. As this recipe makes two loaf cakes, you can freeze one for later.

Put **300g (1¾ cups) yellow polenta (cornmeal)** in a bowl.
Pour on **500ml (2 cups) boiling water** and stir in well.

Leave to cool while you prepare the rest of the ingredients, which can all go in another bowl:
  15g (1 cup) dandelion petals (see p77 for their preparation)
  400g (2¾ cups) ground almonds (we usually grind whole almonds, as we like the nuttier chunks in it)
  1 teaspoon baking powder
  4 teaspoons agar powder
  ¼ tsp salt
  200g (1 cup) golden granulated or light demerara sugar
  finely grated zest of a lemon

Add the polenta mixture to this bowl and then **185ml (¾ cup) olive or melted coconut oil**. It will look as though it's too dry but keep stirring and it will all become moist.

Spoon into two oiled loaf tins. Bake at 175C/350F for 40 to 50 minutes, until it is lightly browning on top.

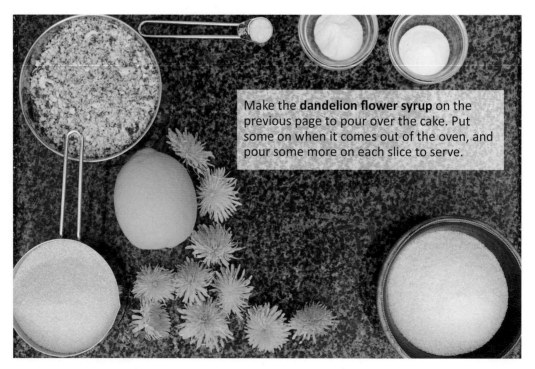

Make the **dandelion flower syrup** on the previous page to pour over the cake. Put some on when it comes out of the oven, and pour some more on each slice to serve.

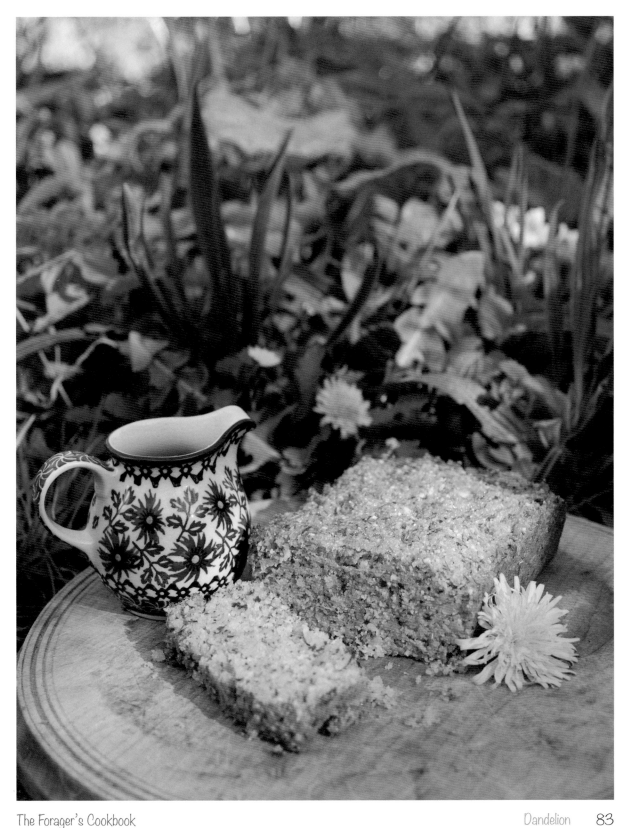

Dandelion Fizz

This is a lovely sunny soft drink which uses the natural yeast found in dandelion flowers to ferment it enough to make the drink fizzy.

Boil **200g (1 cup) sugar** in **500ml (17fl oz) water** to dissolve the sugar.

Let it cool, then add
2 liters (4 pints) water
a colander full of dandelion flowers
an orange, chopped
a lemon, chopped

We make ours in a big glass sweet jar but any large ceramic, glass or stainless steel container will work. Leave it to sit for 3 or 4 days, stirring each day.

Strain out the dandelions and the fruit, and bottle the liquid. Swing-top bottles work well for this. Check for fizz after a day or two. The speed of fermentation depends on the temperature, so your drinks will be ready faster if the room is warm. Once the carbonation is where you want it, store the bottles in the fridge and consume within a couple of days.

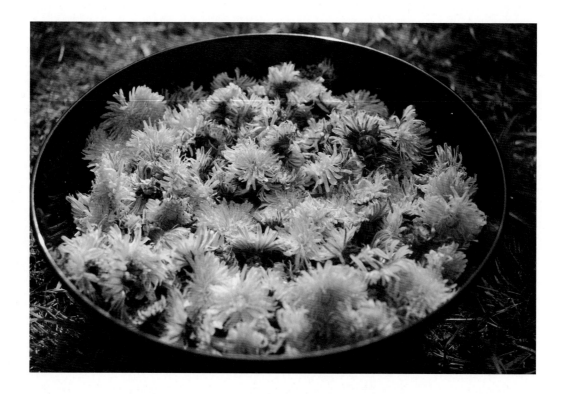

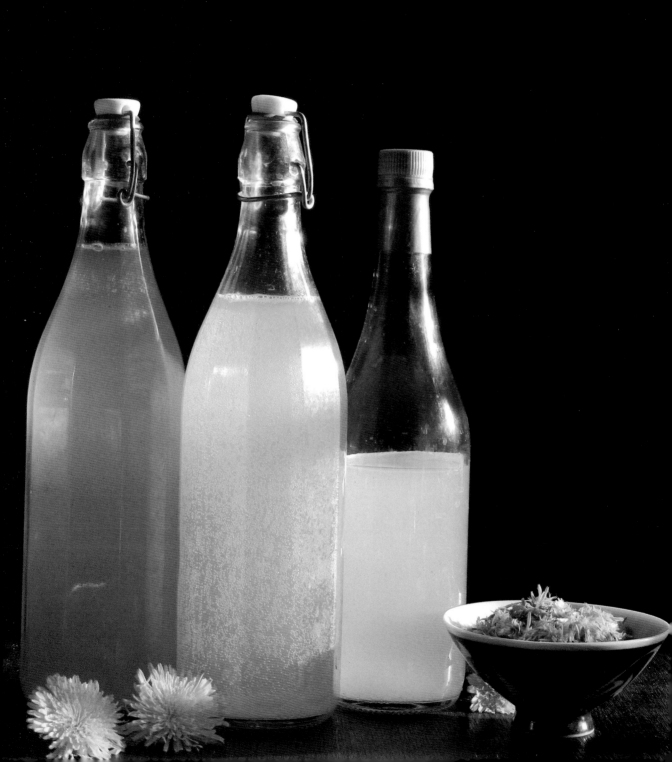

Elder

Elder (*Sambucus nigra*) has made the slow journey from protective mother-spirit to backyard and garden weed, fit only to be sawn down.

We explore these transforming identities, along with others: elder as successful commercial crop, domestic medicine and source of wonderful summer drinks and autumnal puddings and savory beans.

**Adoxaceae
Moschatel family
(formerly in the
Caprifoliaceae)**

Perennial deciduous shrub or small tree.

Edible parts: Flowers in midsummer, berries in early autumn.

Distinguishing features: tree or shrub, according to habitat; branches are pithy, stems hollow; compound leaves with 5–7 pairs of leaflets, pointed, smooth and toothed; flowers creamy-white, with 5 rounded petals and prominent stamens, borne in rounded or flat-topped showy clusters; berries deep purple when ripe; 3 seeds per berry.

Edible relatives: American elder (*S. canadensis*) and blue elder (*S. caerulea*) can be used interchangeably with *S. nigra*; another North American species, red-berried elder (*S. racemosa*), is mainly used for its flowers although the berries can be cooked in jams and jellies.

Cautions: do not ingest the leaves and stems, or eat the berries raw. The raw seeds contain cyanogenic glycosides.

What kind of a weed is elder?

Elder (*Sambucus nigra*) is a deciduous perennial shrub-tree – it can grow to 10m (33 ft) or more when left undisturbed in semi-shade and in a nitrogenous soil, but survives as a man-size shrub in poorer ground or when suffering wind exposure.

It is, these days at least, often considered a weed, to be removed by chainsaw, whereas once it was a sacred tree, Mother Elder.

The classic textbook on weeds by Salisbury (1961) offers two reasons for elder's weedness (as we term it): early, unnoticed growth in winter and speed of shoot development in spring, leading to elder's destructive shading.

In our minds, elder only makes us notice it for six months, from about April to October in Britain and North America, when it is a showstopper, with its panicles of extravagant creamy, fragrant blossoms followed by succulent blue-black fruit.

In winter, though, elder is dishevelled, stark, algae-covered. It is, in the words of plant-journeyer Charlotte Du Cann (2012), *Bony, scraggly, ghost-branched, broken-headed. She* [elder] *is at the end of things, and yet, even in the coldest month, in the winter's depth, small dark-red leaves are sprouting…*

By April the shoots and leaves are full of vigor – the shoots can put on over 2m (7ft) a year. This 'exceptional rapidity', explains Salisbury, causes a shade problem for adjacent shrubs in the yard and garden, and they sometimes fail and die.

The old countryman's belief that elders stunt and poison their neighbors, leading to gaps in the hedge that stock can get through, may originate here.

But there's also a far older Christian myth that elder was the tree of Christ's crucifixion and also where Judas Iscariot hanged himself. The sign of God's displeasure was the twisting of elder's branches and the miniaturization of the fruit.

In other words, the tree was accursed and to be shunned, the worst of weeds.

It all stretches credulity, to be honest. Elder is simply not good at weight-bearing, its brittle stems capable of supporting its large clusters of blossoms or fruits, but not strong enough to be used as a wood.

One student of ours found that he could make sturdy beads from elder stems, and dye them with the berries (for violet and purple), the leaves (yellow) or the bark (grey and black). He was doing what the crofters did, in dyeing the colors of Harris Tweed.

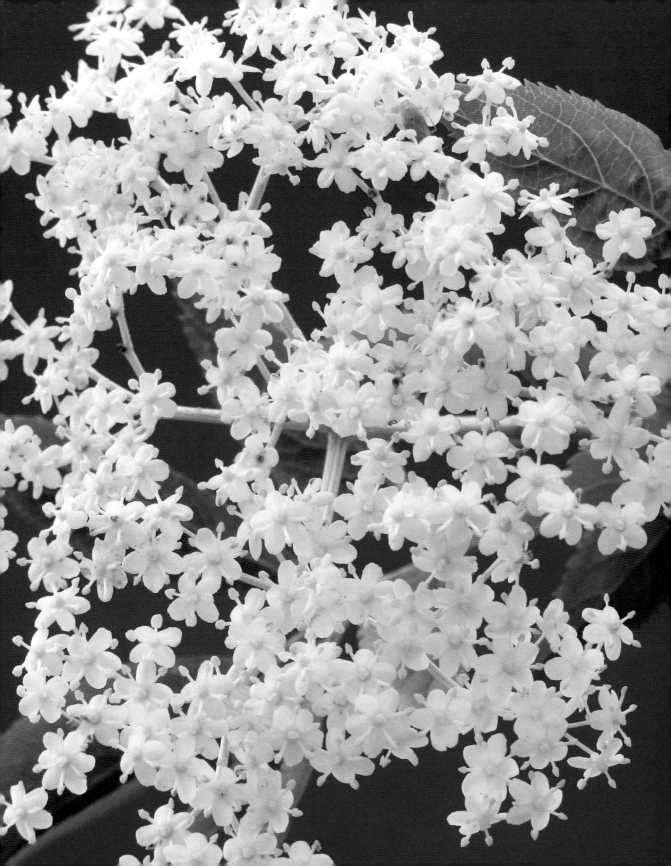

The history of elder

Elder accompanied man as he settled the post-glacial world. Like nettle, elder proliferates where human waste provides it with the nitrogen-rich earth it likes, but it can equally manage without us, as it does near rabbit warrens and badger setts.

Elder spreads mainly by animals and birds swallowing its fruit and excreting the seeds in a new habitat. In addition to suppressing nearby competing plants it has a suckering habit, but lacks aggressive rhizomes.

One early interaction with man arose from the hollowness of elder's stems, which are filled with a spongy pith. A Greek legend has it that Prometheus stole fire from the gods on Mount Olympus and carried the hot coals in an elder stem.

Later, the hollow stems were used as pipes to fan flames. Later still, the Anglo-Saxons gave their name for fire, *aeld*, to elder, perhaps because the pith could be dried as tinder. Elder, however, has never made desirable firewood as its damp core spits and screams – the Devil at work, some say.

Air is another elemental human connection with elder. Finger holes could be pierced in the easily hollowed-out stems to make flutes, whistles or pipes. Indeed, the genus name *Sambucus* was given to elder by the Roman naturalist Pliny the Elder (an appropriate name!) in the first century AD, referencing the flute called a sambuca made from elder stems.

Continuing with former names in remembering ancient wisdoms, Hylde Moer, Mother Elder, was a Scandinavian guardian, sometimes known in English folklore as Old Lady or Old Girl.

It was good fortune if elder planted herself in your backyard (rowan was better in the front), meaning that the Mother had chosen to protect your house, family and animals against witchcraft and unnamed terrors.

It also meant you should pay respects to the elder, never cutting or burning it without praying to the Mother first. Here was elder as sacred tree.

Herbal & other uses of elder

Elder has another, modern identity, that of a commercially successful product. It is one of the few weeds in this book to be grown and harvested for profit in Britain. In England the public has an unquenchable thirst for elderflower cordial and champagne; in North America the berries are in demand, made into jams, jellies and syrups.

The first large British producer of modern times was Belvoir Fruit Farms, in the east Midlands; starting in 1984 with 1,000 bottles of cordial, by 2015 their output was 1.5 million bottles, and growing.

In the US, figures from 2019 indicated a national market worth over $113 million, with notable recent growth in elderberries as a cold and flu treatment sold in mainstream stores.

Elderflower cordial, wine and pressé have long been popular, but more recently elder has been discovered by chefs as a novel flavor for sorbets, fritters, vinegars and gins.

A final identity for elder is as a famed domestic medicine. John Evelyn in 1664 (see quotation on left) considered it a 'catholicon', or cure-all, and he found all parts of the plant useful.

In our times the bark and root are considered rather too purgative for everyday use, but the flowers taken as a tea encourage sweating and help break a fever. The flowers, as a tea, can also cut congestion and relieve respiratory infections and hay fever.

An entry from a Norfolk book of culinary recipes, 1739–79, advises: *Elder flowers dry boiled in milk & drink it at night. It weill sweat & do much good.*

The berries have a positive effect on the immune system and help reduce the severity and duration of winter sniffles.

How to gather and eat elder

Using the flowers: The smell varies with exposure to direct sunlight: in open sun, it is attractively lemony, but in shade can be unpleasantly musky. Sniff before you pick! And don't pick the flowers in wet weather.

Morning picking is a good rule. This might be hampered by elder's thuggy colleagues, nettle and bramble, but because the panicles are large and readily snipped off at the base of the flowerhead (we use scissors rather than tear them), gathering a plentiful harvest can take just a few minutes.

The flowering season, remember, is short, sometimes a couple of weeks. A guideline to optimum picking is to watch the pollinators: on a dry day, the more insects on the flowerheads, the nearer the peak of perfection they are.

A gentle distillation of elderflowers produces a sweet and heady water, while a cold infusion, leaving the flowers overnight to suffuse in filtered water, is equally delightful.

Elderflower water, made by either method, was once used like lavender or orange water to tone the complexion.

The flowers combine well with the flavors of gooseberry, raspberry strawberry and rose in a fruit salad.

The dried flowers retain their potency through until the following year and can be used as a tea.

Using the berries: The unripe berries make good capers, suggest the English forager John Rensten (2016) and US-based chef Pascal Baudar (2016).

The ripe berries are luscious and blend well with sweet spices and most fruits. They contain high vitamin C and blue anthocyanins, and make our preferred syrup for winter coughs.

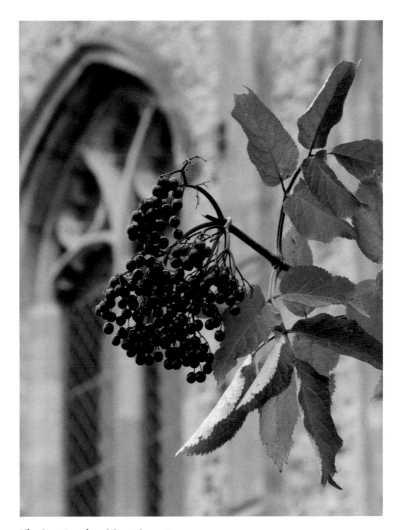

The berries should not be eaten raw; heat them in your recipes, or filter out the seeds from the juice using a muslin bag. The raw seeds can cause tummy upsets or diarrhea.

Gathering the bunches of berries is as straightforward as for the flowers. Some people strip the berries using the tines of a fork, or simply use your fingers. The juice color washes off your hands easily.

The berries freeze well, or if for immediate gratification, they combine well with apple in baked puddings such as crumbles and pies. Or try an elderberry vinegar or spiced beans.

… the easily made and surprisingly pleasant fizzy, summer drink 'Elder-flower Champagne'.
– Wynne Hatfield (1964)

Elderflower & Rose Cordial

Elderflower cordial is delicious, but tastes even better with the addition of rose petals.

Pick 30 heads of **elderflower** on a dry sunny day, choosing those that smell lemony and fresh. Pick **a double handful of rose petals**, preferably from red or pink roses for the color.

Boil **1kg (2lb) sugar** in **2 liters (4 pints) of water** for about 5 minutes in a large saucepan. Pour into a large ceramic bowl and add **50g (2oz) citric acid, a chopped lemon** and **a chopped orange**.

Add the elderflower heads and rose petals. Stir well. Cover with a clean cloth and leave for 3 or 4 days, stirring every day. Strain through a jelly bag and bottle. For long-term storage, the cordial can be frozen.

To drink, dilute to taste with cool sparkling water. It can also be made with hot water to encourage sweating in colds and fevers.

Alternatives: The cordial can be frozen to make a sorbet or poured into popsicle moulds to make ice pops. Extra rose petals can be added to make the color brighter.

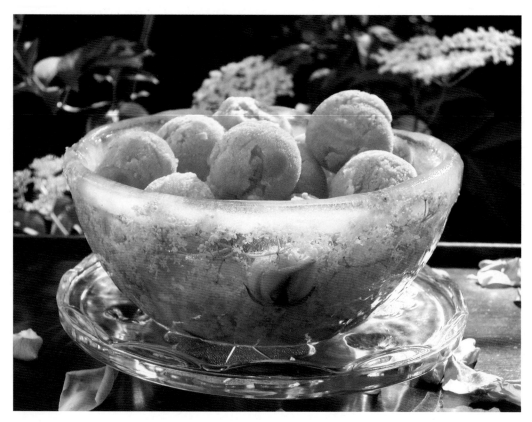

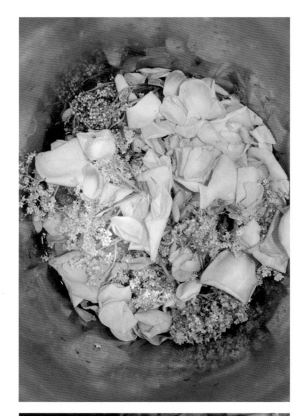

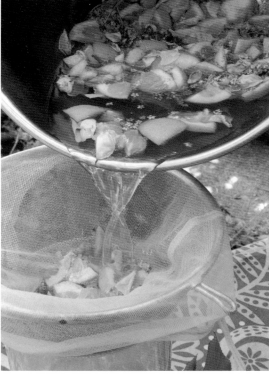

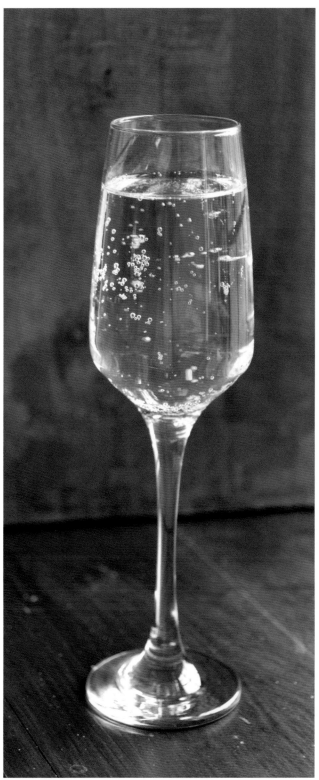

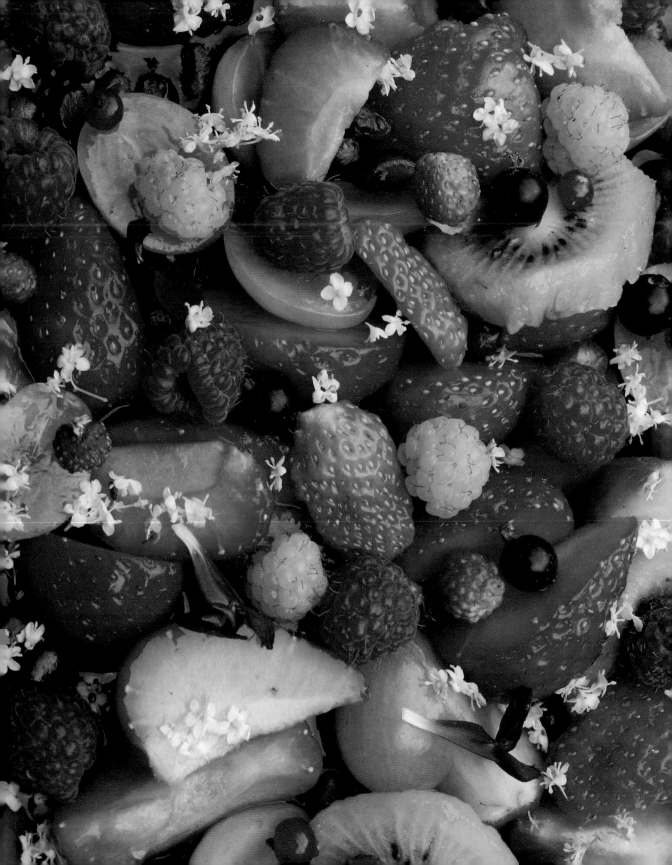

Elderflower **Fruit Salad**

Elderflower combines well with fruity flavors, and can add an extra zing to fruit salads. If the fresh flowers aren't in season, just use the cordial and decorate with whatever other edible flowers are available.

Take a selection of summer fruits such as:

strawberries and wild strawberries
red and yellow raspberries
grapes, cut in half
slices of kiwi fruit
red and blackcurrants
pomegranate

Soak them in some elderflower or elderflower and rose cordial for about 20 minutes, stirring ocasionally to coat the fruit.

Put in a serving dish, along with the liquid, and decorate with **individual elderflowers** and **other edible flowers** such as salvias or borage.

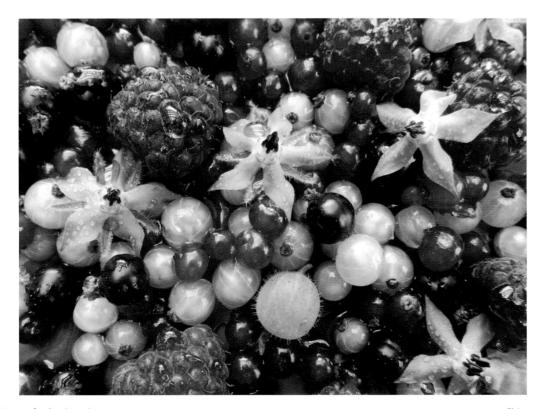

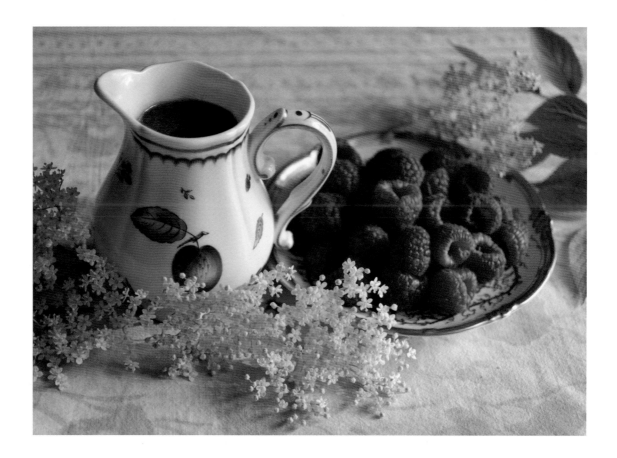

Elderflower & Raspberry **Coulis**

Elderflower and raspberry complement one another perfectly, and the rose in the cordial makes it even more delicious. Coulis goes well with pancakes, ice creams, creamy tarts and cheesecakes. Or serve it with sliced bananas for a simple but delicious dessert.

Put in a saucepan **400g (3¼ cups) raspberries** and **100g (½ cup) sugar**, and heat until the sugar starts to boil and the raspberries go mushy.

Push through a sieve to remove the seeds, using the back of a spoon to press the fruit pulp through.

Add **a tablespoon lemon juice** and **60ml (¼ cup) elderflower and rose cordial**. Taste, and add more lemon if you think it needs it.

It will keep in the fridge for a couple of days, or it can be frozen for later use.

Alternatives: Strawberries can be used instead of raspberries, and of course you can use plain elderflower cordial if you don't have elderflower and rose.

Elderberry **Vinegar**

Elderberry vinegar is a lovely rich red color. A teaspoon a day can be taken to ward off winter viruses and coughs. It can be sweetened or left tangy, and can be used in salad dressings or to add a zing to a variety of dishes. Try combining it with elderflower cordial as a shrub, used like a cordial with sparkling water for a refreshing drink.

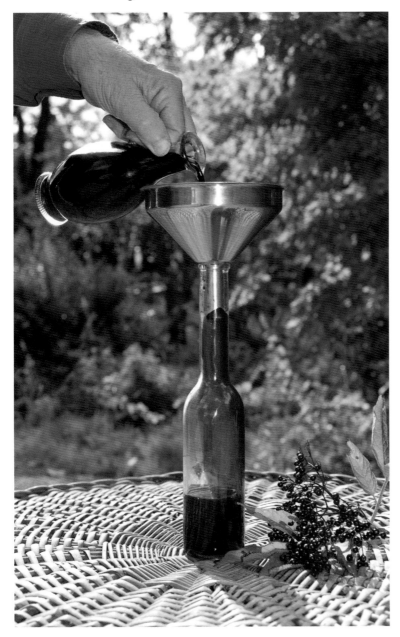

Fill a jar with **elderberries**, stripped off their stalks. A fork works quite well to do this, or you can simply use your fingers. It won't matter if there are little bits of stem left, as you will be straining it once it has brewed.

Pour in **red wine vinegar** to cover the berries. Put the lid on and leave for about a month, shaking occasionally.

Press out the liquid, squeezing to get out as much as possible, then bottle. This should keep in a cool place for a year or more.

Alternatives: If you want to make a quick version, gently heat the berries with enough vinegar to cover them. Don't boil them, as a gentle simmer is enough. After about half an hour, strain off the liquid, and bottle.

The vinegar can be sweetened to taste using sugar. Brown sugar gives a richer flavor but may darken the vinegar.

Other vinegars such as cider vinegar can also be used as a base.

Elderberry Spotted Pudding

This is a traditional steamed pudding adapted from a recipe of Julie's grandmother.

Rub **120g (1 cup) coconut oil**
into **300g (2½ cups) flour**

Add **150g (1 cup) elderberries** and **110 g (½ cup) maple syrup or 300g (1 cup) golden syrup (light treacle), warmed**
Dissolve **1 teaspoon soda** & **a pinch of salt** in **250ml (1 cup) water**

Stir to mix well. The batter will be quite runny.

Pour into an oiled medium pudding basin. The batter needs plenty of room to rise, so the basin should only be about half full.

Tie a cloth over the top – we use a cloth napkin tied on with string – and then fold the corners up to use as handles to lower it into a large saucepan to steam. The water should come about halfway up the sides. Put a lid on the saucepan.

Steam, simmering or gently boiling the water, for 2 hours.

Serve warm.

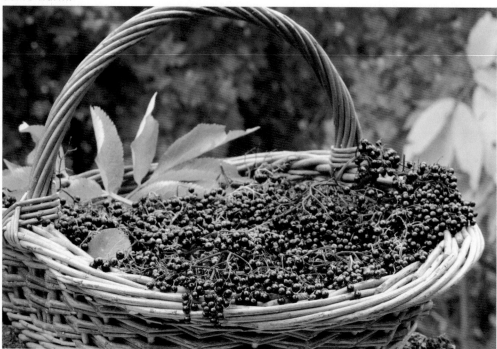

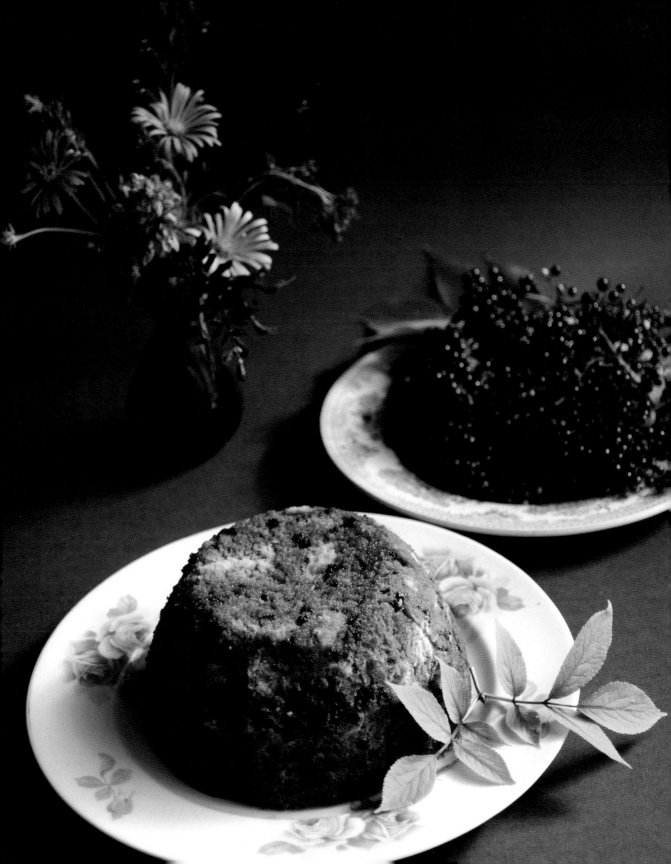

Elderberry **Beans**

We use elderberry juice and cocoa powder in this bean recipe to give an extra richness to the beans. Add more chilli if you like your beans really spicy.

Soak **500g (1lb) dried pinto beans overnight**

Cook **2 onions, diced**, in **a little oil**
Add **2 chillies, finely diced**

Add **1 teaspoon smoked paprika powder** and **½ tablespoon chipotle paste**

Add **500g (2 cups) elderberry juice** and **2 tablespoons cocoa powder**

Add **the drained, soaked beans** and **enough water to cover the beans**.

Put a lid on the saucepan and simmer gently.

After about half an hour, add **75g (½ cup) elderberries** (omit if you don't want the slight crunchiness the berries give), **½ teaspoon cinnamon powder** and **1 teaspoon finely chopped rosemary**.

Continue cooking until the beans are tender, topping up the water if they get too dry.

Add **salt to taste**. Serve with rice or tortillas and a salad.

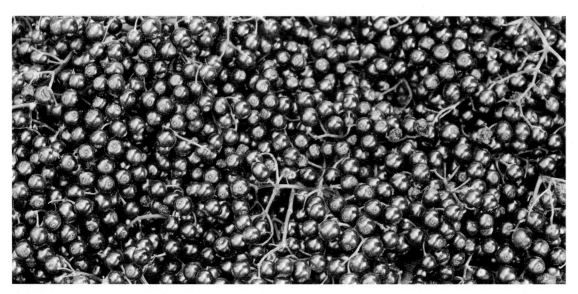

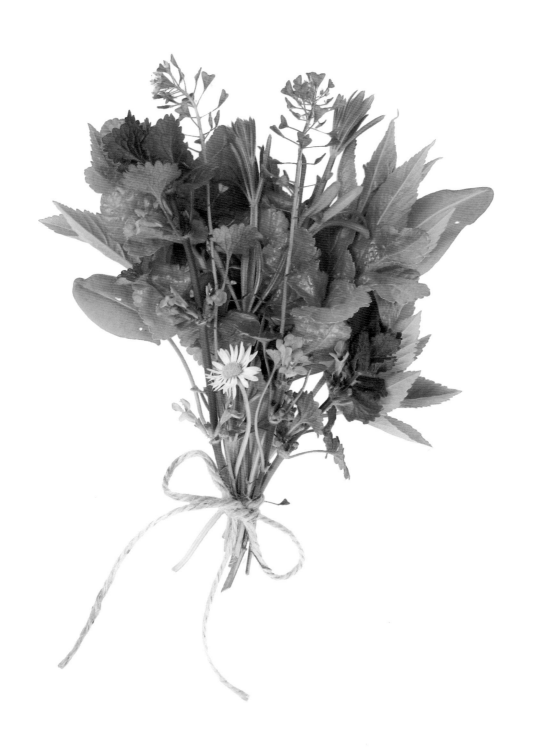

Fat Hen & Orache
(Lamb's Quarters)

You may find it offputting to be invited to eat something once called muckhill weed, but we hope you will give fat hen (and orache) a culinary chance. Blame the medieval arrival of spinach for the decline in their popularity because they remain tasty wild greens. South American relatives amaranth and quinoa are already gluten-free foodie favorites.

Amaranthaceae
Goosefoot family

Annual.

Edible parts: The leaves, flower buds and seeds are picked in summer.

Distinguishing features: The leaves are generally triangular in the *Chenopodiums* (fat hen-like) but thinner and willow-like in *Atriplex* (orache-like) species. Leaf shape can be quite variable, even on one plant. Flowers are tiny and borne in clusters at the tops of the stems.
The whitish-looking appearance of the leaves in some species derives from small hairs catching the light; an alternative name for fat hen is white spinach. Don't worry if you can't identify the exact species, as they are all edible.

Edible relatives: Good King Henry (*Chenopodium bonus-henricus*) is a perennial, as is sea purslane (*Atriplex portulacoides*). Quinoa (*Chenopodium quinoa*) and amaranth (*Amaranthus* sp.) are important food species from South and Central America.

What kind of weeds are fat hen and orache?

We look at fat hen and orache together as probably the most familiar wild weed members of the Amaranth or goosefoot family.

Fat hen, or lamb's quarters in the US (*Chenopodium album*), is a denizen of farmyard and field, flourishing in nitrogen-rich soils and piles of organic waste or middens. Among graphic old names were midden mylies in Scotland, and muckhill weed, dirty dick and pigweed across rural England.

The fat hen name itself probably came from the attractiveness of the flowers and seeds to chickens, and the meat that farmers could derive thereby. In Normandy the name was similar, *la poulette grasse*.

The Latin name translates as white goosefoot. *Album* refers to the white 'mealy' appearance of young plants. Goose-foot is the literal meaning of *cheno-podium*, and is from the basal triangular leaves that are vaguely goose foot-like.

Another farmyard animal reference is the English name lamb's quarters, now the dominant name in North America; mutton chops or mutton tops are other English West Country names.

Orache or arrach (*Atriplex patula*) is a far-travelled and well-mangled English form of the old Greek and Latin names *atraphaxis* and *atriplex* respectively. Confusingly, it has also been called fat hen and lamb's quarters, as indeed the plants are similar in appearance.

This similarity reflects rampant hybridization, with multiple subspecies and varieties named in both plants. The Kew *Plant-List*, a global standard for plant nomenclature, lists over a thousand microspecies of both *Chenopodium* and *Atriplex*; *C. album* alone has 79 entries and *A. patula* has 30. Luckily you don't need to worry about this level of detail to eat them.

Among the many *Chenopodiums* are microspecies names for white, yellow, golden, grey, pallid, green, purple and shiny goosefoots. One is more like a tree: *C. giganteum*, tree spinach, grows to 2m (6.6ft). Our favorite name is *C. detestans*, the New Zealand fish-guts plant, and no doubt the smelliest member of the family.

In botanical terms fat hen shows a 'plastic response' to its environment. This means it readily grows tall and robust in the most nitrogen-rich substrate but is small and 'weedy' in less good soils. We remember finding fat hen in a nutrient-poor sand dune in Ireland, near the Burren coast, flowering at 10cm (4.5in) high.

Fat hen can develop from seed to fruit in 100 days, but takes longer in adverse conditions, another plastic response and a useful survival mechanism.

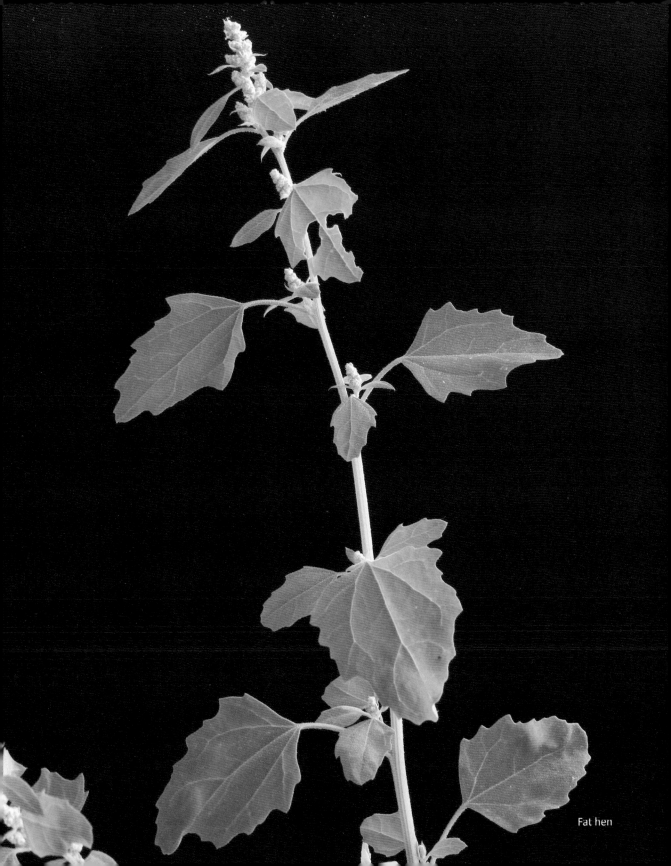

Fat hen

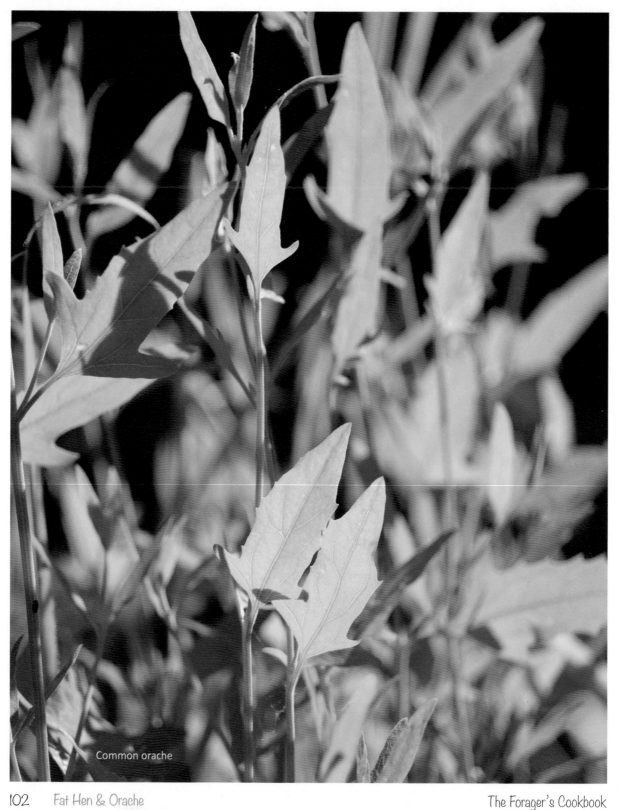

Common orache

Another adaptation by fat hen is that it is allelopathic, meaning it suppresses the germination and growth of competing plants, whether other wild species or farm crops.

As an agricultural weed, fat hen is a significant problem in England for sugar beet and potato crops, though not for cereals. One study showed its presence caused a 48% loss in a sugar beet field. This is ironic as sugar beet is a fat hen relative in the beet family.

In most Australian states fat hen is a declarable hazard for arable crops.

In northern India, by contrast, *Chenopodium* species are cultivated for food – see p111 for our attempt to make *Bathua ka Saag*, a fried green vegetable accompaniment to curries.

It is convenient that exact ID of the goosefoots is not vital when considering them for food. The related species of *Chenopodium* and *Atriplex* are all edible and can be used interchangeably and safely.

The history of fat hen and orache

The oldest record of a goosefoot species is from Bavaria, where 2007 research unearthed fossil remains of *Chenopodium wetzleri* some 28 million years old.

In archaeological rather than geological time, there is evidence worldwide of human use of goosefoot in remains of ovens, storage pits and in cultivated fields. These probably reflect a fraction of the age-old interaction of man and the Amaranths.

Given that the species in focus, fat hen and orache, abound on middens, which accompany any human settlement, these were no doubt significant foraged food items long into prehistory.

It helps that the leaves can be eaten raw or cooked, grow quickly and are nutritious and satisfying; the cooked seeds made for good porridge and a form of unleavened bread.

At times along their co-development with man the farmer, the Amaranths have been cultivated by hand and in small fields, as they still are in rural South America and India.

Spinach (*Spinachia oleracea*) is an Amaranth species that originated in Persia and travelled both west and east in medieval times, soon being preferred as a vegetable to the goosefoots and beets. China is now the spinach-eating center in the world.

Fat hen and orache seeds have a possible future role as gluten-free 'pseudo grains', similar to the now readily available amaranth and quinoa.

All along the Amaranths have been valued as food but also vilified as weeds. The plants are just surviving and thriving where they can, and it is human perception and priorities that render them heroic or villainous.

All the same, if a field of sugar beet is full of its weedy relative fat hen, nature might be telling us what we ought to be thinking about growing there.

It reminds us of a recent true story we heard from the supervising gardener at the Islamic garden in the new Cambridge Central Mosque.

Fat hen was flourishing in the disturbed ground of the site. A number of Pakistani ladies who were clearing the site were overjoyed to see such familiar weeds, which they quietly gathered to take home and cook.

Herbal & other uses of fat hen and orache

Underlying their dense nutritional capacity, the leaves of both plants are high in vitamins A and C, and when the seeds are added, supply all the ten amino acids necessary for human functioning.

Medicinally, a tea made from either plant is somewhat astringent, and can be a gentle mouthwash. As a home remedy it will ease upset stomachs,

[fat hen is] *very wholesome medicine, as well as a pleasant vegetable, and an excellent substitute for spinach.*
– Grieve (1931)

They [fat hen] *are probably the best wild leaves for eating, with a flavor reminiscent of kale and young broccoli. Use the leaves and tender tops, discarding the tougher stalks.*
– Carluccio (2001)

Lamb's-quarters is one of our best wild potherbs. It has a delicious taste, is easy to find, and deserves to be better known and appreciated.
– Silverman (1997)

[Orache is] *much more palatable than* [fat hen], *with leaves high in Vitamin C that were used to bolster up the clear soup given to convalescents. It is very easy to grow and deserves greater popularity.*
– Barker (2001)

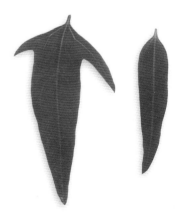

Leaf variation in orache: two leaves from the same plant

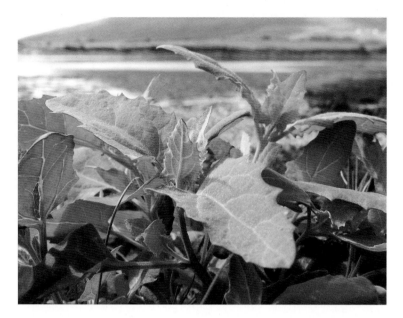

Young fat hen growing by the sea, The Burren, Ireland

Fat hen with roots, center front, on a market stall in Munnar, south India

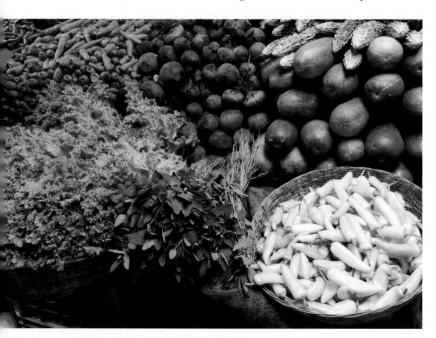

The fat hen relative **epazote** (*Dysphania ambrosioides*), also called Mexican tea, herba sancta Mariae and wormseed, was once 'official' in the *US Pharmacopoeia* as a treatment for roundworm, including in children.

Epazote was sold commercially in essential oil form as 'Chenopodium oil' and was also advised for hookworm and tapeworm for dogs and humans. Human trials indicate that the active principle in epazote, ascaridol, combats multidrug-resistant tumor cells. Epazote is strongly antifungal and antioxidant, and in trials protected stored wheat from fungal attack.

Fat hen too has been demonstrated to suppress cell growth in human breast cancer cell lines, suggesting a novel way to make positive use of the plant's allelopathic quality.

In South African folk medicine the leaves of epazote are burned and the smoke inhaled to treat mental disorders and convulsions (i.e. it is spasmolytic).

Note that large and repeated quantities of epazote are potentially toxic and can stimulate menstruation and even unplanned abortion. Fat hen and orache, by contrast, are non-toxic.

How to eat fat hen and orache

Both plants are easy to collect, and the leaves and flowerbuds can be stripped from the fibrous, inedible stalks without the hazard of thorns or prickles. We found it slow work, though, to collect leaves for our *Bathua* recipe, taking 40 minutes for 400g.

The leaves cook quickly and retain their flavor; nor do they go bitter with age through the growing season. The usual cautions apply about not gathering your leaves where there may be contamination.

Blanching or boiling the leaves is sometimes urged so as to neutralize any oxalic acid content. People with kidney issues should thus be cautious in using the leaves raw in salads.

relieve gas and may soothe diarrhea. In previous times the leaves were recommended for use against scurvy.

Externally, the same tea can be applied on insect bites or stings, or for nettle rash. In India a tincture of fat hen is rubbed into rheumatic and arthritic joints. The family's old reputation for being a laxative can also be put to use.

Fat Hen Freekeh Salad

Put in a saucepan together **100g (½ cup) freekeh**, **250ml (1 cup) boiling water** and
¼ teaspoon salt.
Cook for 25 minutes, or until the water has all been absorbed.

Leave to sit for a few minutes, while you make the dressing:
Put in a blender **60ml (¼ cup) olive oil,**
             25ml (½ cup) citrus juice (juice of an orange and a lime)
             1 clove garlic
Blend until smooth.

Add **25g (1 cup) chopped fat hen or orache leaves**
Shake to mix well
Add to the warm freekeh
Add **150g (1 cup) chopped cherry tomatoes**

Alternatives: Try adding pomegranate seeds and thin slices of kumquat. If you need to
make a gluten-free version, use **300g (1½ cups)** cooked quinoa instead of the freekeh.

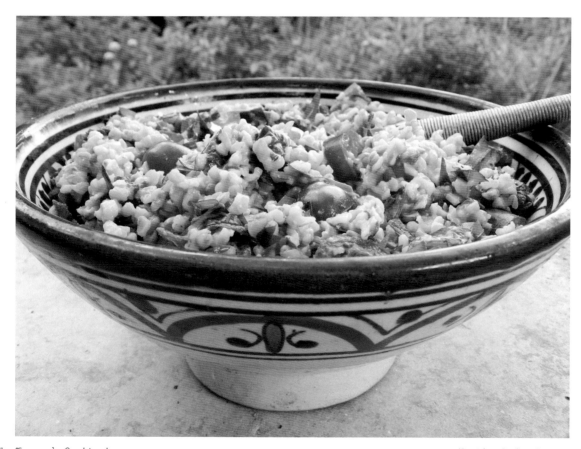

Orache Tart

We usually make this tart with a combination of orache and fat hen but have called it orache tart because we usually have more abundance of orache in our garden, and the leaves are very pretty for decorating the top.

Lightly **oil** a flan dish. Pour some **sesame seeds** into the dish and turn to coat the bottom and up the sides as your base – just as you would to flour a greased cake pan. Tip out the excess, though you can leave a thicker layer in the base of the dish if you wish. Preheat oven to 180C/350F.

Put in a blender:
- **280g (2 cups) raw cashew pieces**
- **30g (¾ cup) gram flour** (or chickpea/garbanzo flour)
- **500ml (2 cups) water**
- **1 tablespoon oil**
- **1 or 2 cloves of garlic**
- **1 teaspoon chipotle paste or smoked paprika**
- **½ teaspoon salt**
- **½ teaspoon turmeric powder**

Leave to sit while you sauté **2 onions, chopped.**
When the onions are turning translucent, add about **140g (2 handfuls) of fat hen and orache leaves, chopped**.

Continue cooking until the leaves have wilted and turned a deep green.

Pour about half of the cashew mixture into the bottom of the dish, then spread the vegetables on top, and cover with the remaining cashew mixture.

Decorate the top with leaves if you want a wow factor.

Bake for 30 minutes, until the flan is set. Remove from oven and allow to cool for a few minutes before serving.

Alternatives: Instead of the sesame seed crust, you can use hulled hemp seeds; or a blend of soft sun-dried tomatoes and ground nuts pressed into the pan; or you can use a normal pastry shell. Ground elder leaves and sow thistle are also good in this recipe.

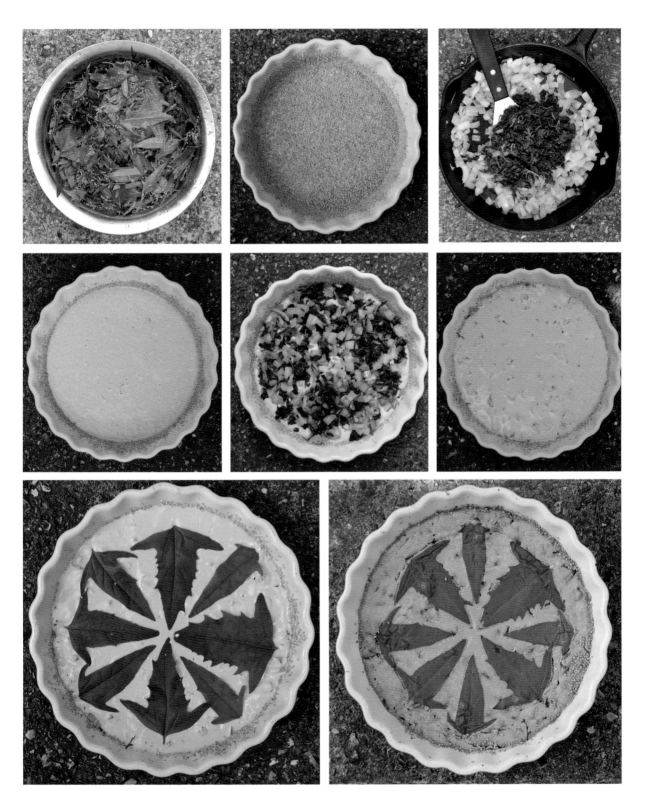

Fat Hen **in Coconut Milk**

This recipe is inspired by palusami, a well-known dish from Polynesia where greens, usually taro leaves, are cooked with coconut milk.

Finely dice **an onion**, then sauté in **a little oil**.

Add   **1 or 2 cloves garlic, crushed**
               1 tablespoon finely grated ginger
               350ml (1½ cups) coconut milk
               about 100g (3½ oz) fat hen and orache leaves, chopped coarsely
               1 or 2 teaspoons white miso

Stir and cook until the leaves are done, then add:
               juice of a lime

Serve with rice and toasted coconut flakes. Serves 2.

Alternatives: If you don't have lime, use lemon juice instead.

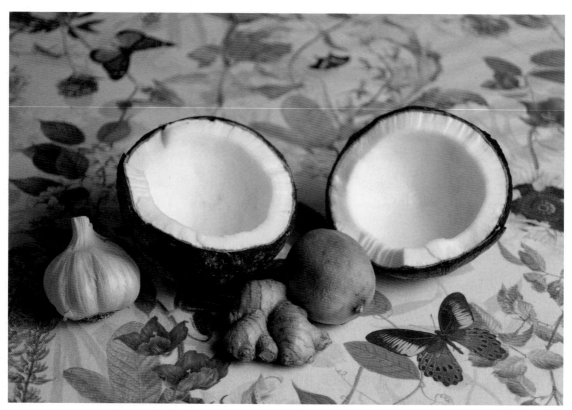

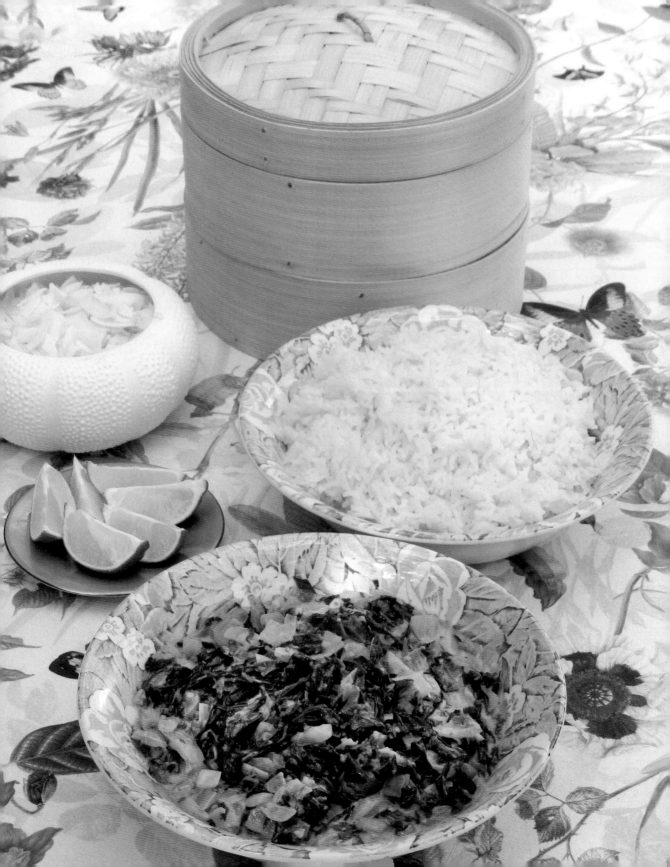

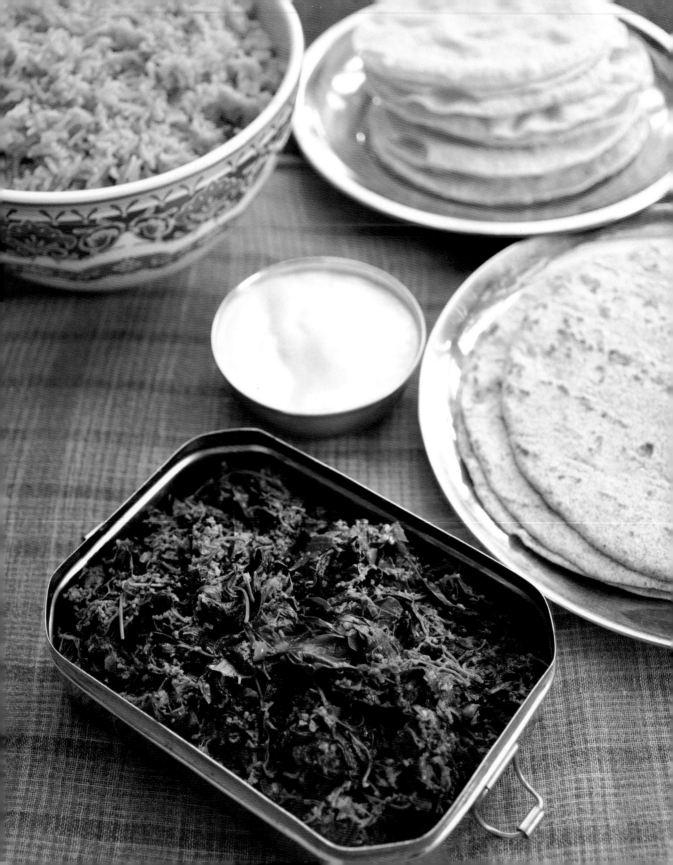

Bathua ka Saag

Bathua ka saag is a popular North Indian dish that is a delicious way to prepare fat hen and orache. In northern India, fat hen grows best in the cooler winter months, but in most of Europe it will be a late summer crop.

Every family has their own recipe, but the basic idea is the same. Many cooks will use more oil than in our recipe, but this version is suited to our taste. If you prefer a smooth consistency the leaves can be puréed in a blender, but we find that they are so tender that this isn't necessary.

For this recipe you'll need **a colander full of fat hen and orache leaves & flower buds, or about 400g**. Remove the leaves and flower buds from the stalks – this is the slow part! Wash the leaves and flower buds in water, then blanch in boiling water for about half a minute. Rinse in cold water.

In a large saucepan, heat on medium heat **2 teaspoons mustard oil or sesame oil**

Add   **1 teaspoon cumin seeds**
           1 teaspoon mustard seeds
When the seeds begin to splutter, add
2 large cloves garlic, crushed

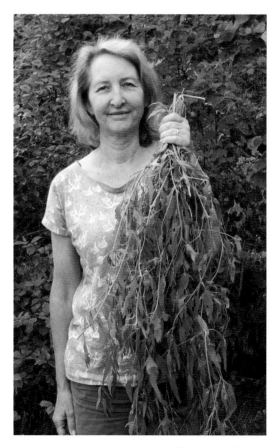

Cook for about a minute, then add
1 or 2 green chillies, or to taste, finely chopped and the blanched fat hen and orache leaves.

Cook over low heat with the lid on. Stir occasionally until the leaves are tender – 10 to 15 minutes. The leaves should still be damp enough from rinsing, but add a little water in case of sticking.

Add **salt to taste**.
Serve warm with chapatis or paratha and rice.

Alternatives: You can vary the spicing to taste, for example by using turmeric, coriander or fenugreek.
Onion can also be added.

Julie holding a large orache plant, freshly harvested, which gave 125g stripped leaves

Fat Hen Empanadas

These delicious pastries are perfect for picnics, as an appetizer or for lunch.

Preheat the oven to 200C/390F.

Gently fry a **chopped shallot or onion** in **a little oil** with **a clove of garlic, minced.**

When the shallot has turned translucent, add **100g (½ cup) cooked chickpeas (garbanzos).** Continue frying for a few minutes, then add **200g (a cup) of cooked butternut squash or pumpkin, cubed.**
Then add a large handful **(½ cup) of chopped fat hen** and **2 spring onions (scallions), chopped.**

Continue cooking for a couple of minutes, then set aside to cool.

Roll out **a package of short crust pastry** to about ¼ cm (⅛ inch) thick, and cut out circles of about 10cm (4in) in diameter. Put a tablespoonful of the filling in the center of each circle, wet the outer edges with **a little water** and fold in half. Crimp the edges by pleating with your fingers or press them with the tines of a fork to seal.

Place the finished empanadas on a baking sheet and bake for about half an hour, until golden brown.

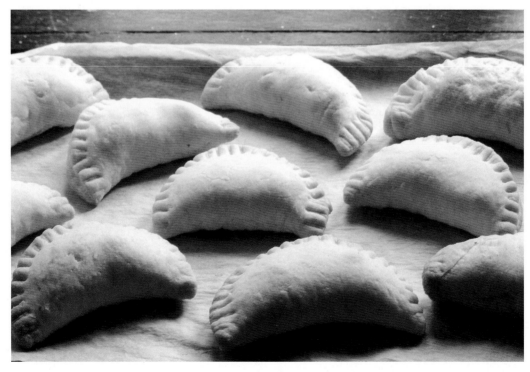

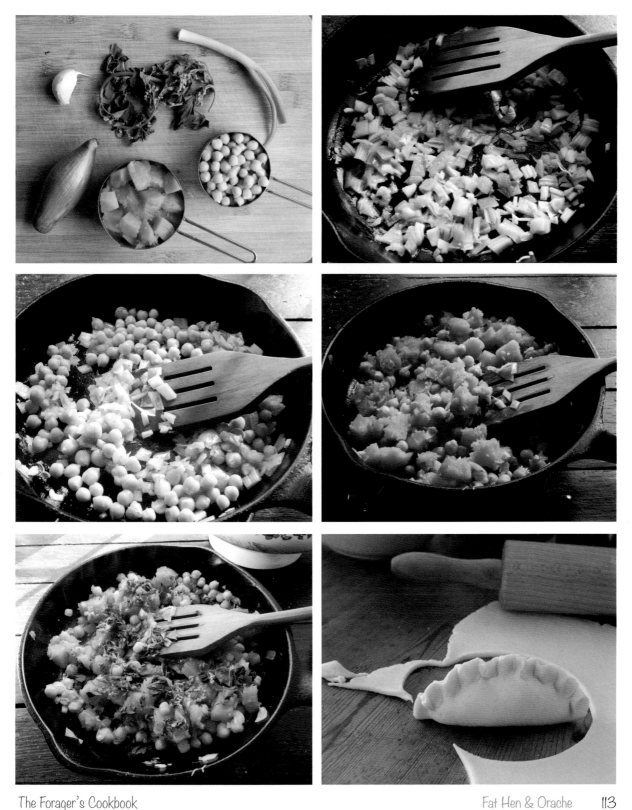

Ground Elder

Ground elder (*Aegopodium podagraria*) is one of the weeds that gardeners most love to hate. It spreads everywhere and is virtually impossible to get rid of. But if you can't beat it you can at least eat it! The young bronze-colored leaves have a fresh but strong taste, like a gentle version of lovage. Our recommendations include the raw roots and shoots, cooked bhaji, frittata, 'bishop's delight' and a mild kimchi mix.

**Apiaceae
(formerly Umbelliferaceae)
Carrot family**

Perennial. Leaves die back in winter, and resume growth in the spring.

Parts eaten: Leaves, year round but especially in spring when they are young and shiny. White rhizomes.

Distinguishing features: Dark green low-lying foliage, the undivided, pointy leaves resembling the elder tree (no relation); slender, hairless and hollow stems; handsome white cow parsley-like flowers in summer at about a meter (3.3ft) tall; beige roots and white, spear-like rhizomes; forms dense colonies.

Edible relatives: Several wild members of the carrot family, e.g. alexanders, wild fennel, pignut, sweet cicely.

Photo opposite: the ultra-white flowers of ground elder are fine and delicate for a 'thug' of a plant, and are well set off by cornflowers

What kind of a weed is ground elder?

One summer the local village gardening group came to visit our garden. We had told them we had a sort of forest garden of herbs, weeds and flowers. Don't expect tidy rows, we said, and we will talk about foraging in your own backyard.

The group was happy to hear about the virtues of dandelion and daisies, thistles and nipplewort, and nibble on the odd leaf or two. And then it came to ground elder (*Aegopodium podagraria*).

Weeds are clearly one thing but ground elder another, a superweed, a demon presence. Tasting its young leaves – a fresh, strong flavor, they agreed – hardly appeased the good folk, and accusations of gardening insanity were not far away.

Then we offered them our ground elder filo pastry rolls. That stopped the muttering in its tracks. These are really rather tasty, one person said. Is there another one?

The moral of the story is that getting behind the conventional can open up new debates, new considerations.

If the leaves are young enough, they taste good; and the more you pick the more new tender leaves you will have. This is the secret of backyard foraging: keep eating your weeds when they are small and you will have a perpetual supply of fresh, tasty greens.

Back to the original question, slightly rephrased: what makes ground elder so successful? We identify three factors, each powerful.

First must come its roots. In addition to its regular beige-colored roots, ground elder has white rhizomes, in the form of thin, spear-like runners. These are fast-spreading (up to a meter a year) and indomitable.

They can lance horizontally through the roots of any other plant, entangling with them and making it impossible to weed and transplant the victims.

The runners sprout their own thin roots and can resurface a few inches or feet away from the mother plant as a clone. It is a highly effective form of vegetative reproduction and is why you get colonies of ground elder in the form of total ground cover.

But these white runners can be collected and eaten like bamboo shoots in some token fightback for the takeover of your land (see p118).

The second factor in the unstoppable spread is that, unfortunately for gardeners, ground elder can regrow from the smallest slither or fragment (i.e. it is apomictic). Digging it up in effect serves to spread it, as does filling

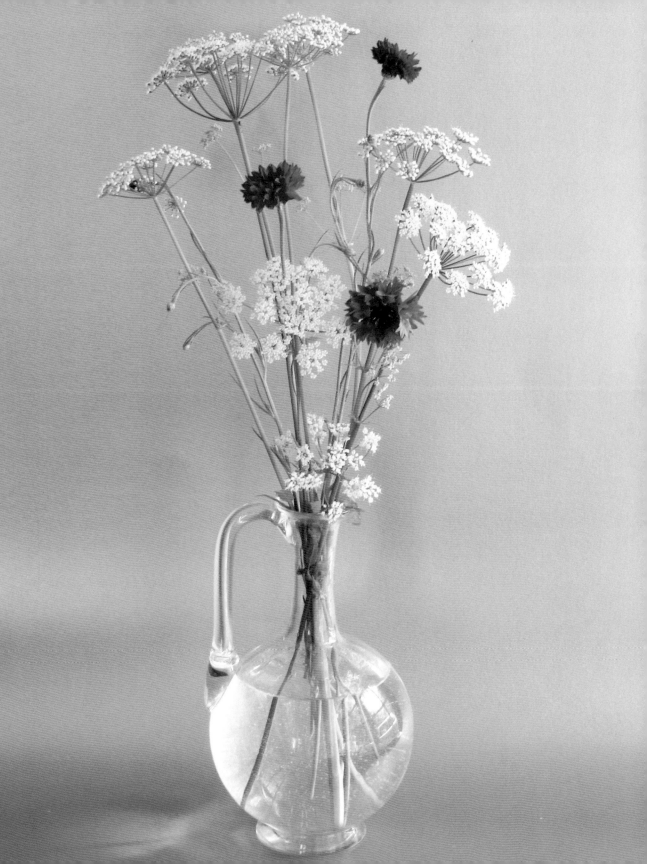

your compost heap inadvertently with ground elder-rich soil.

Matthew's mother refused to accept any plants from our garden because we have a ground elder presence. It's that bad, with even your own mother (sensibly) turning away your random acts of filial kindness.

Thirdly, ground elder reproduces itself in the normal way too – an old name is jack jump-about. If you let your plants flower, though, you may be surprised at how handsome the pure white flowers are, and they look fantastic in flower arrangements. Picking them will stop the seeds spreading.

It doesn't help the gardener in us that ground elder tolerates a good deal of shade and poor soils, and it also dries out the soil below it.

The history of ground elder

It is moot whether the Romans brought ground elder with them from southern Europe to Britain. The archaeological record hasn't yielded a definitive answer, and we don't know whether the Romans might have eaten the plant, used it for medicine or introduced it by accident.

In any case by medieval times ground elder was a familiar presence in British monastic gardens. It was grown not for food or for pleasure but as a hard-working medicinal, as its old common name of goutweed reveals.

Another old name is herb Gerard, after St Gerard of Toul (935–994), patron saint of gout sufferers. The species name *podagraria* also means gout.

Gout is a painful condition of the joints in which uric acid gathers as crystal deposits, particularly in the big toe. The condition can be related to excessive indulgence in alcohol and rich food, inspiring another old name, bishopweed.

The higher clergy were long known for over-use of port and fine wine, and suffered for it. But drinking ground elder tea or eating the leaves, perhaps placing a poultice on the affected joint, reduced the pain by helping the body dissolve the crystals.

In one instance a revered religious figure was said to have enjoyed eating ground elder. The Russian saint Seraphim of Sarov (c1754–1833) secluded himself in a forest hut and ate mainly ground elder for three years.

Old monastic foundations, broken up nearly five hundred years ago, still have thriving patches of it, as we saw one summer when visiting the grounds of Llanthony abbey in the Black Mountains of south-east Wales.

The global expansion of ground elder was probably accidental via the presence of its root fragments in soil containing desired flowers or crops, though in Victorian parks and botanic gardens there are examples of deliberate planting as ground cover.

It is seldom planted at all nowadays, though variegated versions are sometimes sold in garden centers.

In Sweden you can buy ground elder as a delicacy in supermarkets, while in Norway the extreme gardener Steven

Ground elder is named for the similarity of its leaves to elder

Elder

Barstow, author of *Around the World in Eighty Plants*, founded a social media group called Friends of Ground Elder. We are duly among the small group of FOGE, making a case for revenge eating.

The rest of the world, strangely enough, has remained immune to the charms of ground elder, and it has become a global villain of the temperate garden. It is officially an invasive weed in parts of North America, especially the northeast, and Australia.

Gardeners know well to avoid adding the rhizomes to the compost pile, and that you shouldn't allow it to seed – ground elder spreads quite sucessfully without any help from us. The flowers are beautiful, however, and can be used in flower arrangements. They hold their petals better than cow parsley.

Herbal & other uses of ground elder

Gout treatment by ground elder is familiar, but the plant is a useful backyard remedy for inflammation generally, penetrating and soothing swollen areas with the same lance-like efficiency as the rhizomes underground. It has also been used to relieve rheumatism and sciatica.

It is specifically valuable for problems and imbalances of the kidney and urinary system, taken as a tea or externally soaked in a poultice.

Modern research on rats is supportive of traditional findings of ground elder normalizing uric acid metabolism, and being anti-inflammatory and protective against carbon tetrachloride-induced hepatitis.

Another animal research finding is that it has hypoglycemic qualities that are potentially beneficial in human metabolic syndrome treatment.

How to eat ground elder

Most people seem to have a bad initial experience of nibbling ground elder

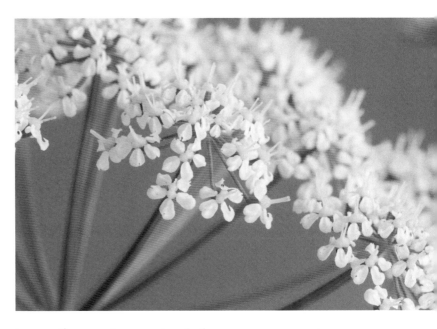

because they are given a mature leaf to try. These, we find, are too strong in flavor and only palatable if well cooked.

The shiny fresh young leaves, on the other hand, are nutty and tender. These make good eating raw or cooked, as do the young flower stems. Older stalks are too fibrous to be enjoyable, but the young ones can be stripped of any woody outer layers and cooked, for example, as a pasta substitute.

You can take control of ground elder's growing season by continuing to harvest young leaves and stems of the plant, for almost a year-round harvest.

The white rhizomes too can be picked at most times, but spring is best. Their taste and appearance are reminiscent of bamboo shoots.

It takes us about 20 minutes to fill even a regular cupful, and it was curious to see that some small plants had a good supply of the rhizomes while some larger-foliaged plants had none.

There is no short cut to rhizome gathering, but it helps a little to remember you are weeding as well as gathering dinner.

I wouldn't do without it as a vegetable and I use it frequently in spring over a 6–8 week period when the fresh young growth is available. I also use it later in the summer where it regenerates the areas where it still grows in my forest garden.
– Barstow (2014)

Ground Elder Roots & Shoots

Ground elder, as you will know if you have it in your garden, spreads by white underground rhizomes that will force their way through so-called weed-proof membranes and most other barriers. The good news is that they are tasty to eat, crisp and juicy – a bit like a bamboo shoot. Use the younger white ones, as the older light brown ones get tough.

They can be added to stir fries at the end of cooking, or try a tasty salad of rhizomes and very young leaf shoots. A light dressing of mirin and toasted sesame oil is all they need.

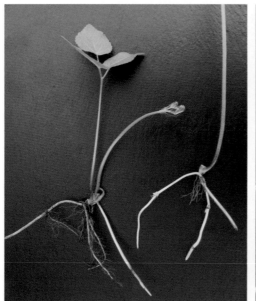

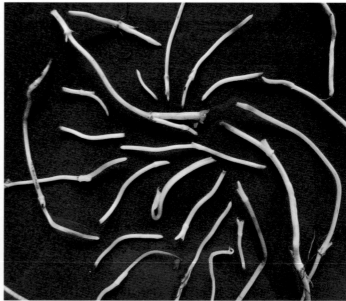

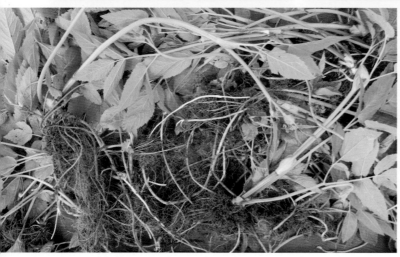

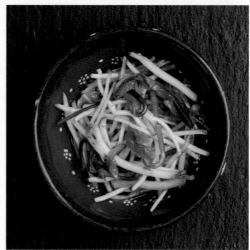

Ground Elder **Bhajis**

We don't eat much deep-fried food in our house, but these are a firm favorite as a treat. They are a tasty snack at any time, but also an ideal starter for an Indian meal. And they are gluten-free!

Mix: **250ml (1 cup) water**
140g (1½ cups) gram flour (or chickpea/garbanzo flour)
½ teaspoon salt

Add: **30g (1 cup) chopped ground elder leaves**
150g (1 cup) chopped onion
1 teaspoon turmeric powder
1 teaspoon cumin seeds, crushed

Deep fry in hot oil (at 190C/375F), a tablespoonful at a time.

Drain. Serve with lemon wedges and a salad.

Alternatives: Any of the leafy greens in this book could be used in this recipe.

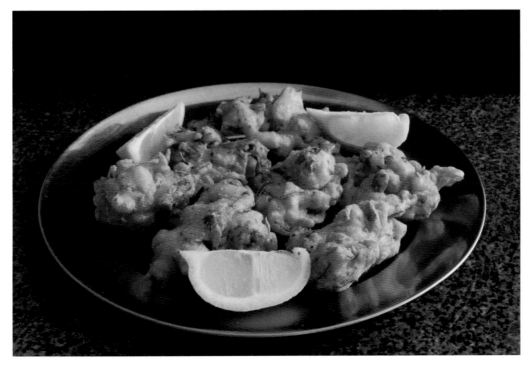

Ground Elder **Frittata**

This vegan frittata can be made with all sorts of wild greens, but ground elder has become our favorite. And if you have ground elder in your garden, you probably have plenty of it!

Preheat the oven to 175C (350F).

Put in a blender:
- **1½ cups water**
- **80g (¾ cup) gram flour** (or chickpea/garbanzo flour)
- **30g (¼ cup) raw cashew nut pieces**
- **1 or 2 peeled cloves of garlic**
- **1 teaspoon turmeric powder or 2cm (1in) fresh turmeric root**
- **¼ teaspoon salt or black salt**

Blend until smooth, then set aside while you sauté the vegetables.

Put **1 to 2 tablespoons oil** in a cast iron skillet (ours is 22cm/9in diameter).
Add **a couple of handfuls of sliced mushrooms (about 80g)**, fry until beginning to brown, then add **a couple of handfuls of chopped ground elder leaves (20 to 30g)**. Stir until the leaves have wilted.

Then pour the mixture from the blender over the vegetables, continuing to cook until the edges of the batter begin to set, then transfer into the preheated oven.

Bake for about 15 minutes. The fritatta should be set, and gently browning on top.
Cut into wedges and serve warm. Serves 2 to 4.

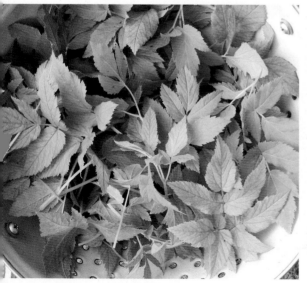
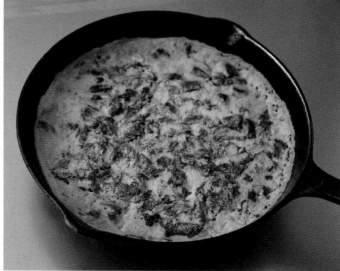

Ground Elder **Bishop's Delight**

This recipe makes 8 small filo pastry rolls. Preheat the oven to 190C/375F.

Pick **about 100g (3–4 cups) young ground elder leaves** (the tender lime green ones) and remove from the stalks. Boil briefly to soften, then drain, cool and chop.

Mix with:
    50g raw cashews, coarsely ground
    2 tablespoons white miso paste
    ¼ teaspoon nutmeg powder
    Add **a little water** if needed to make the mixture hold together.

You will need **4 sheets of purchased filo pastry**.
Take 2 sheets of filo pastry and oil one of them lightly before putting the other one on top. Lay the sheets with the long side towards you, and cut into 4 vertical strips of about 12cm (4.5in) wide.
Take ⅛ of the filling mixture, enough to make a 1cm (½in) roll at the bottom of each pastry strip, leaving 1cm (½in) free at either side. Fold the bottom over the filling, then fold in the sides to make a 1cm (½in) double layer at the edges, and roll up. Brush with a little oil.
Set on a baking tray, and repeat to make the other rolls.

Bake for about 10 minutes, or until golden. Best served warm, they are also good cold.

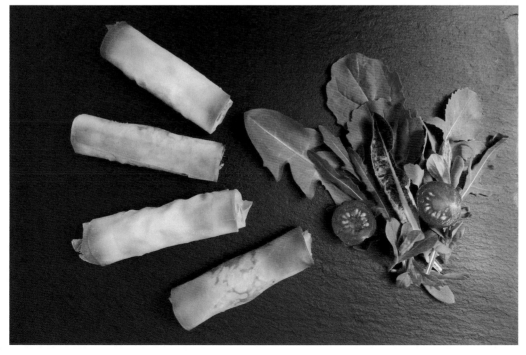

Ground Elder **Kimchi**

This recipe is much milder in heat than Korean kimchi, but you can ramp up the heat if you want to. We used a fermenting jar to make this batch, but we found a large French press or tea press works really well, as you can press the vegetables down below the surface of the salt water without needing a rock.

Put in a large bowl:
500g (1½ cups) sliced cabbage (with a little kale)
100g (3 cups) chopped weed greens (we used mostly **ground elder**, with some chicory, dandelion, sorrel & curly dock)
1 apple, grated

Make into a paste, either with a stone grinder or in a food processor:
1 onion
7 cloves garlic
1 tablespoon paprika
1 tablespoon ancho chilli flakes

Using clean hands, mix the paste and the vegetables.

Mix:
1 tablespoon sea salt
500ml (2 cups) spring or filtered water

Put the vegetables in a wide-mouthed jar, fermenting jar or your French press. Pour the saline mixture in, and stir to let out any air bubbles.

If you are using a jar, put a large edible leaf or two on top – vine leaves or mallow leaves work well, or use cabbage. This can be weighted down with a small clean rock to keep the vegetables submerged. If you are using a French press or tea press, you can omit this step, and just push the plunger in far enough to submerge the vegetables below the level of the brine.

Leave for a few days, tasting each day until the flavor has developed as you like it. The taste will get stronger with time, but some of the freshness of the ingredients will disappear, so this is very much a personal preference. Once you are happy with the fermentation, transfer your kimchi to the fridge.

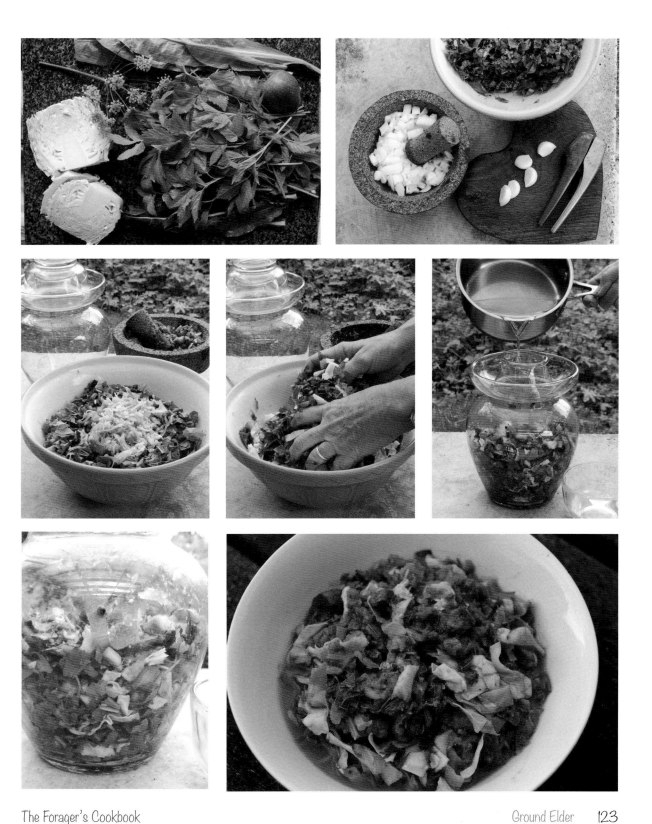

Ground Ivy

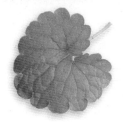

Ground ivy (*Glechoma hederacea*) is both a vilified weed and an appreciated spring wild flower. It has been important medicinally and for a thousand years was an essential ingredient in ale-making. Add to this its subtle and satisfying taste as a tea, and you have the makings of some interesting wild recipes, including scones, buns and kombucha.

**Lamiaceae
(formerly Labiateae)
Mint family**

Perennial.

Edible parts: All above-ground parts; best in spring when flowering, but leaves stay green all-year round.

Distinguishing features: An aromatic creeping, ground cover plant that prefers shady places, under hedges or trees. The square stem and strongly lipped flowers are characteristic of the Mint family.
Flowers appear in early spring, and are usually magenta to light purple, but we have seen a variety with larger pale pink flowers. Leaves are rounded or heart-shaped with rounded lobes, dark green and slightly hairy.

Edible relatives: Woodruff or sweet woodruff (*Galium odoratum*) is used to flavor drinks.

What kind of a weed is ground ivy?

In mid-April, England's roadsides and its less manicured gardens are empurpled with wild flowers as red deadnettle, cranesbills, herb robert and honesty display their full blossom.

Ground ivy is in its prime too. Its color palate, ranging from light lavender or rosemary to deepest blue-violet on the UV spectrum, is highly attractive to insect pollinators.

It is common in fields, gardens and woodland edges across Eurasia from Ireland to Japan, and as an introduced species in North America.

The first American herbal, written by John Josselyn in 1672, records ground ivy as already abundant. It had been brought in by the early settlers to America, for its medicinal and brewing value, and is now an unwelcome invasive in both the east and the Pacific coast.

The naturalist Henry Thoreau spotted it (calling it gill-go-over-the-ground) at Cape Cod in 1865, along with the other imported wild flowers yellow dock, lemon balm and hyssop.

Ground ivy is normally about 15cm (6in) high, but can be double this in conditions of optimal soil and shade. What should really be measured is its width, with the stolons (underground runners that set roots) being often a meter (3.3ft) long.

It is these stubborn ivy-like forms, recognized in the ivy-like name *hederacea*, though there is no link with ivy as such, which create the mat of ground cover over bare earth that leads to ground ivy being dismissed as an unwelcome weed by gardeners and farmers alike.

Evocative older English common names reflect its spreading habit: robin-run-up-the-hedge, blue runner, devil's candlestick, creeping charlie and runaway jack. Additionally it's hard to pull up and will reproduce from the smallest piece left after weeding.

In botanical terms ground ivy is close to the catmints, or Nepetas, and was once called *Nepeta glechoma*. We find its musky scent similar to that of deadnettles, another close relative, and pleasantly pungent. Herbalist William Fernie in 1897 called it 'balsamic'.

We have found the smell becomes subtle, spicy and deeper in cooking. In some places, like the garden of a friend of ours, the ground ivy plants he has are always sweet-smelling.

We mentioned that ground ivy is an invasive weed in North America. In 2011 the self-sufficiency magazine *Mother Earth News* polled some 2,000 gardeners about their worst weeds. Ground ivy came in at no. 6, behind dandelion (no. 2) and chickweed (no. 5). No. 1 was crabgrass (*Digitaria sanguinalis*), in the Poa grass family.

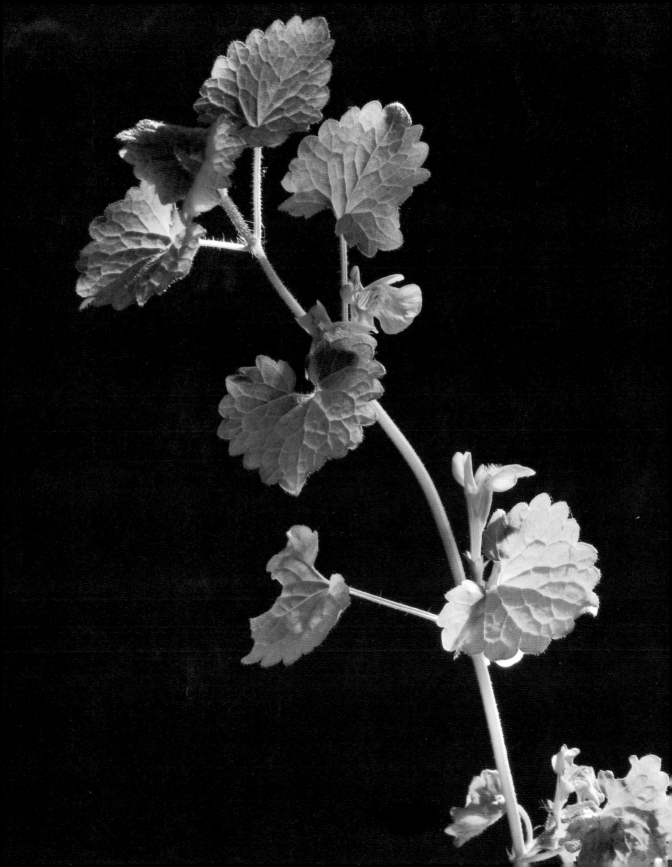

The history of ground ivy

The pan-Eurasian distribution of ground ivy signifies its success since the last Ice Age, over the last 12,000 years and more, in colonizing freshly exposed and warming patches of earth across the northern hemisphere.

There are few archaeological records available, however, to support this remarkable journey or to confirm the plant's original source area.

One exception is a well at the Wilsford Shaft, Amesbury, Wiltshire, excavated in 1989, which revealed the waterlogged remains of *Glechoma hederacea*, in the company of about 100 other wild plants. It was dated to the later Bronze Age, up to 3,500 years ago.

What such finds mask rather than reveal is why a specific plant is within the assemblage. Was it a food or a medicine? Was it abundant or even dominant, or a stray presence with no connection to human use?

On safer ground, we know that the Greeks of about 2,000 years ago named the plant 'Glechoma', meaning mint-like; the classification still holds, and ground ivy remains in the Lamiaceae (mint or deadnettle) family.

Other ancient names, alehoof and tunhoof, highlight ground ivy's role in brewing ale.

The first written use of 'tunhofe' is given in the *OED* online as about the year 1000, from one of the Saxon leechbooks (medical recipe book). 'Alehoue', a variant of alehoof, is recorded as later, from around 1400.

For several centuries, until hops started to be introduced from Germany in the early 1500s, England was an ale country. Ground ivy was a popular bitter plant, as were bog myrtle (sweet gale), heather, yarrow and others, added to malt in ale-making.

Gill ale remained on sale even as hopped beer became the top tipple, as the attached quotations from Dr Quincy and Jonathan Swift illustrate, but by the twentieth century its thousand years of universal ale-making were over.

In 1903 *The American Botanist* sounded its death knell: *Sometimes we call* it [ground ivy] *alehoof, a word equally quaint and smacking of the home brewed and brown draught of merry England.*

Herbal & other uses of ground ivy

Our watchword for ground ivy is clarity. In brewing, it clarifies ale; as a beautiful pale-green tea, it acts for us as a spring cleanse, and helps clear the congestion of a head cold or soothes coughs and upset stomachs.

The German abbess-composer-herbalist Hildegard of Bingen (1098–1179) gave ground ivy in a broth or puree to *a person who languishes, and whose reason is failing; the patient should eat it often, with meat or small tarts.*

Hildegard was renowned for using ground ivy to treat tinnitus. She advised that the plant be boiled in

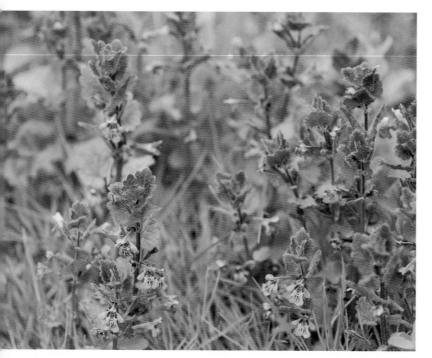

water, the water squeezed out and the wet plant tied to the head as a poultice.

She recommended the same process for chest pains. Again a clearing action is at play.

In ancient Greek and Roman medicine ground ivy was used for eye conditions. To John Parkinson in 1640 it was a 'sovereign remedy' (meaning unsurpassed) for a*ll the paines, rednesse, and watering of the eyes of both man and beasts.*

In France, Jean Palaiseul (1973) describes, rather graphically, how in the days of cockfighting, a cock receiving an eye wound might be dealt with by the owner chewing up a couple of ground ivy leaves and spitting the juice into the cock's eye for rapid healing, and getting it back into the pit.

In France, the same author continues, ground ivy tea was regularly taken for bronchial catarrh, asthma and whooping cough. But it is also a diuretic, as the American forager 'Wildman' Steve Brill once found out.

He describes (1994) having a date with a woman living a few miles away. They picked ground ivy and made tea. He then cycled home. From one cup of tea, he said, he needed to make five pit stops; but there were no pits.

Another story of ground ivy's clarifying action was told by the botanist John Ray in the late 17th century and repeated in later herbals. A Mr Oldacre suffered an 'inveterate head-ach', which was cured by snuffing the juice of the plant up his nose.

A long-forgotten use for the plant was to treat the poisoning suffered by those using lead paint; their complaint was called 'painter's colic'.

The moral for today is that roadside ground ivy could absorb diesel particulates from vehicle exhausts. This means care should be taken to wash the leaves carefully or avoid picking too close to the highway.

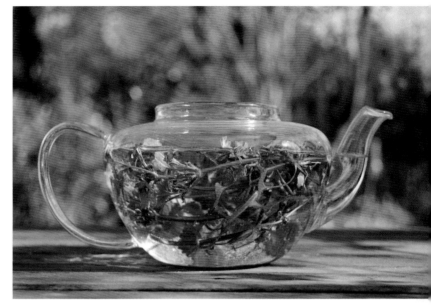

How to eat ground ivy

The easiest way to appreciate ground ivy is as a simple tea or tisane. Gather two or three flowering plants, using all the above-ground parts, and rinse them thoroughly.

Put into a small teapot or saucepan, and pour boiling water over the plants. Allow to steep or brew for up to 10 minutes. Keep a lid on the saucepan so that the vapours do not escape.

The chartreuse-green, and very clear, liquid is satisfyingly salty-sweet, and the musky smell has vanished. It is a delicious spring-cleanse tea in its own right and should be appreciated more.

This can also be your fortified liquid used in baking, as stock for soups and stews or a syrup for alleviating stubborn coughs. Or try it in our kombucha recipe on the next page.

Bushcraft experts Ray Mears and Gordon Hillman (2007) add ground ivy to a nettle soup for 'a bit of bite'.

It is interesting that the flavor of ground ivy works well in sweet as well as savory dishes, leading us to undertake some enjoyable experiments, as we share with you overleaf.

I went to Tooke to give him a ballad and dine with him, but he was not at home: so I was forced to go to a blind [i.e. unnamed] chophouse, and dine for ten pence upon gill-ale, bad broth and three chops of mutton; and then go reeking from thence to the first minister of state.

– Jonathan Swift (1710)

The dealers in ground ivy – otherwise ale-hoof – fought hard against the 'weed' [i.e. hops] which ultimately drove their wares out of the market.

– *All Year Round* magazine (1876)

Ground Ivy **Kombucha**

Ground ivy tea can be used to make a beautiful, fragrant, light golden kombucha. Kombucha SCOBY (that is, symbiotic colony of bacteria and yeast) forms a flat layer on top of the liquid, very like a vinegar mother.

A jar like that shown opposite, with a tap near the bottom, works well. You can turn the tap and remove the liquid without disturbing your SCOBY. When your SCOBY gets to be around a centimeter thick (half an inch) you can give bits of it away to friends who want to make kombucha. It is quite fibrous, so you can also dry it to make a leather-like fabric.

It really freed us up when we learned that you can make Kombucha with herb teas, and don't have to include any green or black regular tea.

Kombucha SCOBY is quite widely available now, but you don't actually need a chunk of it – you can just use a little live kombucha liquid, and it will soon grow its own SCOBY.

So for each **liter (35 fl oz) of cold ground ivy tea**, you will need about **50g (¼ cup) sugar** – we like to use a light unrefined sugar such as demerara. Add about **60ml (¼ cup) live kombucha liquid or a piece of SCOBY.** Cover your jar with a piece of clean cloth, which you can tie on with string or fix with a big rubber band. Kombucha needs to breathe.

Your drink will be ready after a few days, or if the weather is cold it may take a week. Taste after a couple of days, and then each day until you are happy with the flavor balance. It should no longer be too sweet, but not have yet become sharp and vinegar-like.

It can be drunk straight away, but if you'd prefer a slightly fizzy version, pour the liquid into swing-top jars and allow it to ferment gently for another day or so. Once it becomes as fizzy as you like it, keep the bottles in the fridge and 'burp' them now and then – just gently open to let excess carbonation escape.

Kombucha is very easy once you get into a rhythm of starting a new batch once a week or so. Just save a little of the liquid each time for your next batch until you get a healthy-looking layer of SCOBY covering the top of your liquid.

It's very forgiving, or at least the culture we were given is. If your liquid gets to taste like vinegar by being left too long, just pour it into a saucepan and sweat it down over a low heat until it is reduced by about half, then sweeten to taste with a little maple syrup or sugar. When cool, bottle it and use in cooking and for salad dressings – it's a bit like a light balsamic vinegar.

You can get all sorts of wonderful flavor combinations, depending what herb teas you use for the original kombucha.

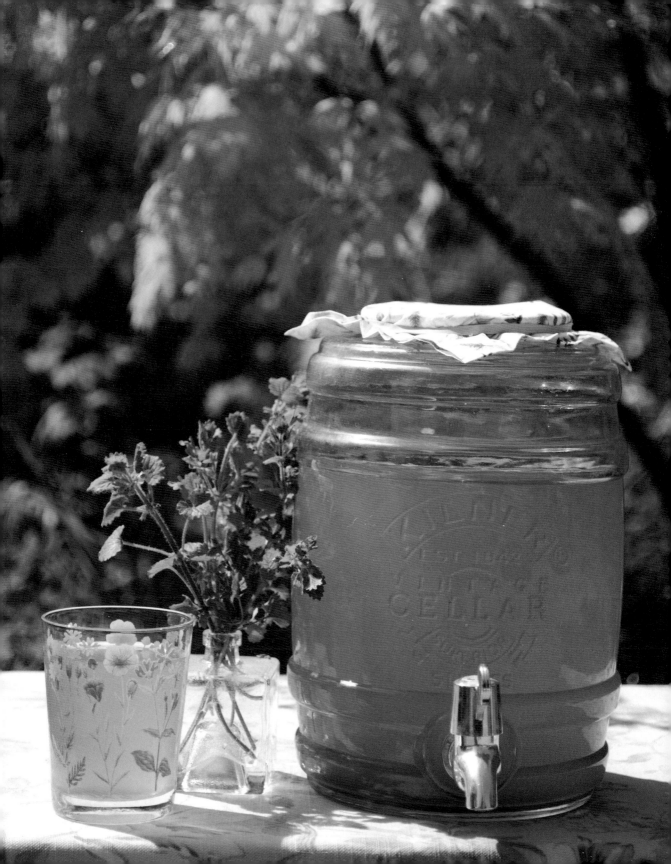

Ground Ivy Hot Cross Buns

Ground ivy is the perfect flavoring for hot cross buns as it is flowering at Easter.

Put in a bowl: **50g (½ cup) raisins**
50g (½ cup) sultanas
3 tablespoons chopped candied peel
225ml (1 cup) strong ground ivy tea
Cover and leave to soak.

When tepid, add: **1 tablespoon active dry yeast**

Add: **240g (2 cups) spelt or wheat flour**
2 tablespoons oil
pinch of salt

Stir until well mixed, then set aside to rest for ½ hour (or overnight in refrigerator).

Knead on a floured surface for about 15 minutes. Cut into 6 or 8 even-sized pieces, and pinch underneath to make round rolls, placing on a baking sheet pinched side down.

Leave in a warm place to rise until doubled.
Brush with **soy milk** to glaze, then bake at 175C/350F for 10 to 15 minutes, until golden brown on top.

While the buns cool, make the ground ivy icing.
Put in a small bowl: **1 tablespoon finely chopped ground ivy**
and pour **1 tablespoon boiling water** onto it.
Cover and leave for about ten minutes, then strain.

To the liquid, add   **2 teaspoons lemon juice**
1 teaspoon finely grated lemon zest

Gradually add enough **icing sugar (confectioner's sugar)** to make a pipeable icing, about ½ cup. Put the icing in a piping bag and ice crosses onto the rolls when they have cooled completely. If the icing is still too runny, put the piping bag in the fridge to cool for a few minutes.

Decorate the icing cross on top of each bun with a **ground ivy blossom**.

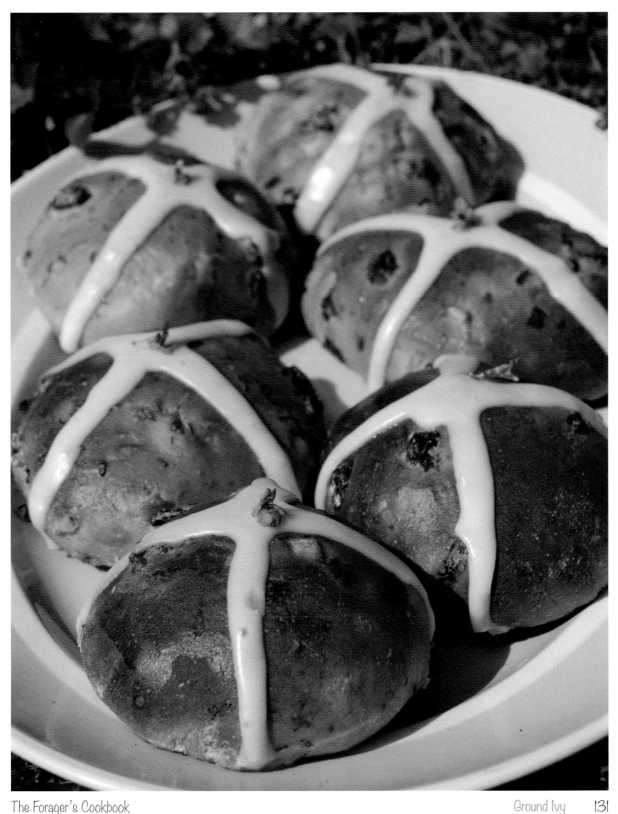

Ground Ivy Scones

These are savory scones, but ground ivy works equally well in sweet scones – simply add a tablespoon of sugar to this recipe.

Rub together until like breadcrumbs:
100g (1 cup) grated cold coconut butter
½ teaspoon salt
2 teaspoons baking powder
1 tablespoon chopped ground ivy leaves
240g (2 cups) flour

Slowly fold in **cold water** with a fork until the mixture is all moistened and will hold together in a soft ball – you'll probably need just a little over half a cup, depending on the flour. On a generously floured surface, press the dough down into a round about 1-inch thick. Cut the dough into circles and place on a well greased and floured baking sheet.

Bake at 200C/400F for about 12 minutes, until a light golden color on top.

Serve with nettle or other soup, or as part of an afternoon tea.

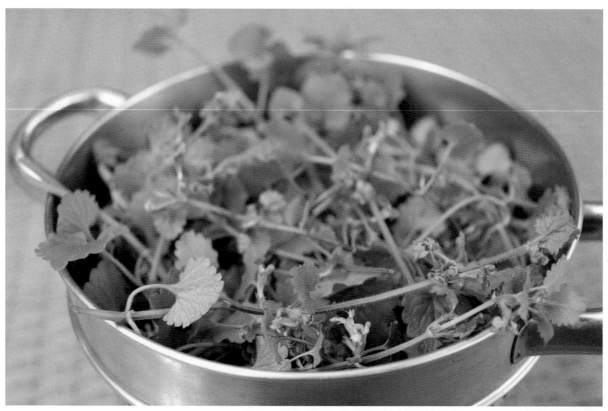

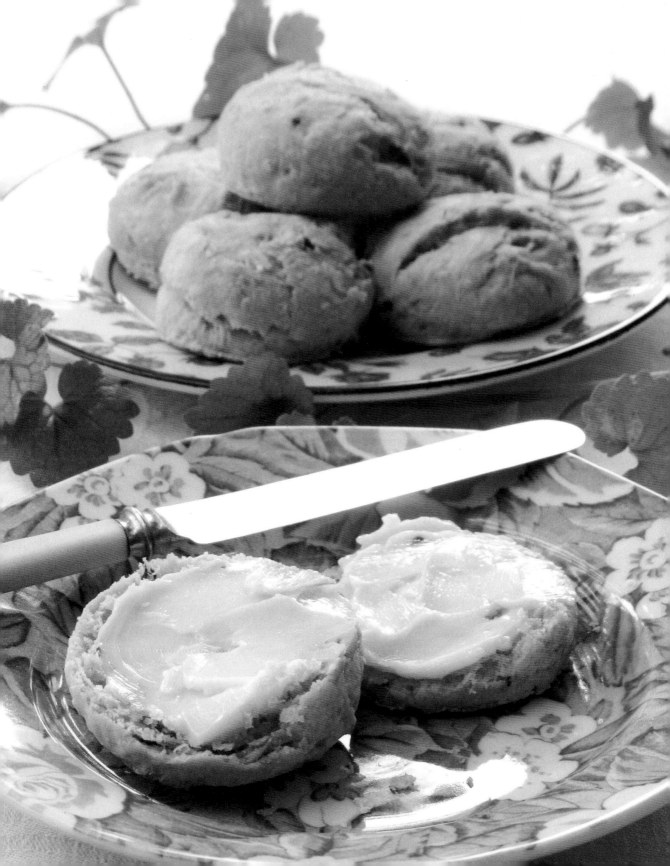

Ground Ivy **Shortbread**

For fun we sometimes call this recipe GI Shorts. Ground ivy gives a wonderful delicate flavor to the shortbread. We use golden granulated sugar, which is crystallized like white sugar but not refined.

Put in a food processor:
70g (⅓ cup) sugar
240g (2 cups) white spelt or wheat flour
115g (1¼ cups) plant butter, cold, cut into small chunks
1 to 2 tablespoons ground ivy, finely chopped

Pulse just until combined.

Press into a 23cm (9in) diameter pie dish or cake pan.

Bake at 165C/325F for about 30 minutes, or until it just begins to turn golden.

Leave for 5 minutes before cutting into wedges. Leave to cool completely before removing from pan.

Alternatives: Yarrow leaves also make a tasty and pretty shortbread – strip the tiny fernlike leaflets off the main stem.
The dough can be cut into circles or other shapes about ½cm (¼in) thick, and cooked on a baking tray. The smaller pieces will need less baking, so check after 15 minutes.

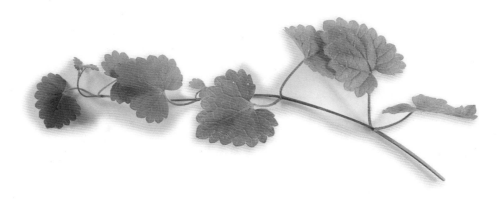

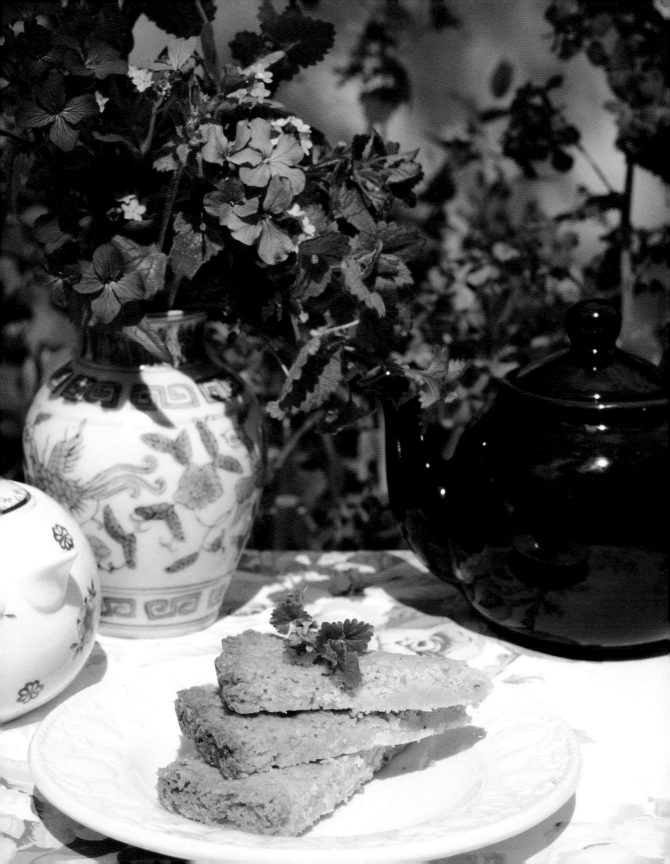

Hogweed (Cow Parsnip)

Hogweed (*Heracleum sphondylium*) is one of our favorite edible weeds, providing a range of flavors through the seasons. It is a common roadside and garden presence, not to be confused with the rare giant hogweed, which is notorious for causing skin blisters. Hogweed provides the iconic winter umbels so beloved of artists, and the flowers are feasted on by a variety of insects. The young leaves, flower buds and flower stalks are all edible, but avoid getting the sap on your skin in hot sunny weather.

**Apiaceae
(formerly Umbelliferae)
Carrot family**

Biennial to perennial.

Edible parts: Young leaf shoots in early spring, flower stalks and buds in late spring, dried seeds in summer or autumn.

Distinguishing features: This is a hairy plant, unlike many others in the family. Flowers in umbels (umbrellas) are creamy white, sometimes pink, with longer petals towards the outer edges. Stems are stout, lime green or sometimes purple, hairy and hollow; to 2m (about 6ft 6in) tall; leaves are broad, deeper green, palmate, rough and usually round-lobed; ovoid, flat green seeds ripening to brown.

Cautions: Hogweed contains furanocoumarins, as do parsnips, angelica and citrus peel. Some people are more sensitive to furanocoumarins than others. Avoid getting the sap on your skin, especially in hot sunny weather, as phototoxicity can cause blistering.
The citrus-flavored bitter green seeds can be nibbled but some people react to them. The ripe brown seeds are safe to use as a spice.

What kind of a weed is hogweed?

Anyone who lives through a northern hemisphere summer will come across hogweed (*Heracleum sphondylium*), one of the commonest of wild plants and weeds. It grows in massed, untidy yet eye-pleasing colonies of frothy cream umbels along lanes and streets, in woods, in fields and gardens.

But is hogweed the same as **cow parsley**? No, they are two different species, close relatives in the Apiaceae (carrot) family. Cow parsley is smaller and less robust, with delicate feathery leaves; it flowers in May, earlier than hogweed, which usually is in peak flower in late June.

Continuing the ID questions, which are imperative to address in the carrot family, is hogweed the same as **cow parsnip**? The answer is 'almost'.

Victorians in England knew hogweed as cow parsnip, but the latter name is now almost only used in North America. There, it refers to a close relative of hogweed, the native cow parsnip, *Heracleum maximum* (or *H. lanatum*), also called Indian parsnip.

Hogweed and cow parsnip are similar, though the latter is generally bigger. American herbalist Michael Moore (1979) called cow parsnip *a large, conspicuous, pleasantly gross plant*.

Hogweed and Giant Hogweed

People often worry about confusing hogweed and its notorious relative, giant hogweed (*Heracleum mantegazzianum*), introduced from Europe to the UK and North America. This can cause serious skin damage, but you can tell the species apart.

Hogweed can be very tall, peaking at about 3m (10ft), but giant hogweed is truly a giant, reaching up to 6m (20ft) tall. Its white flower heads are the size of dinner plates.

Giant hogweed is usually found in damp places, such as along riverbanks. It grows very fast, so the chance of mistaking a young plant for hogweed is slim. Look around for last year's dead stalks near young plants to see which hogweed it is.

Giant hogweed stalks can be up to 10cm (4in) thick, whereas hogweed stalks rarely exceed 2cm (0.8in) in thickness. Giant hogweed stalks are nearly always spotted or blotched purple or dark red, while hogweed stalks are green or uniformly purple. Both are ridged and hollow, with hogweed stalks uniformly hairy, and giant hogweed most bristly at the leaf joints.

Giant hogweed leaves are shiny, hairless and sharply serrated, and can reach 2.5m (over 8ft) in length. Hogweed leaves are from 15 to 60cm (6 to 24in) long, and are not shiny but softly hairy with broad and inflated leaf bases.

For a good guide to ID with photos, see: https://www.wildfooduk.com/articles/giant-hogweed-identification/

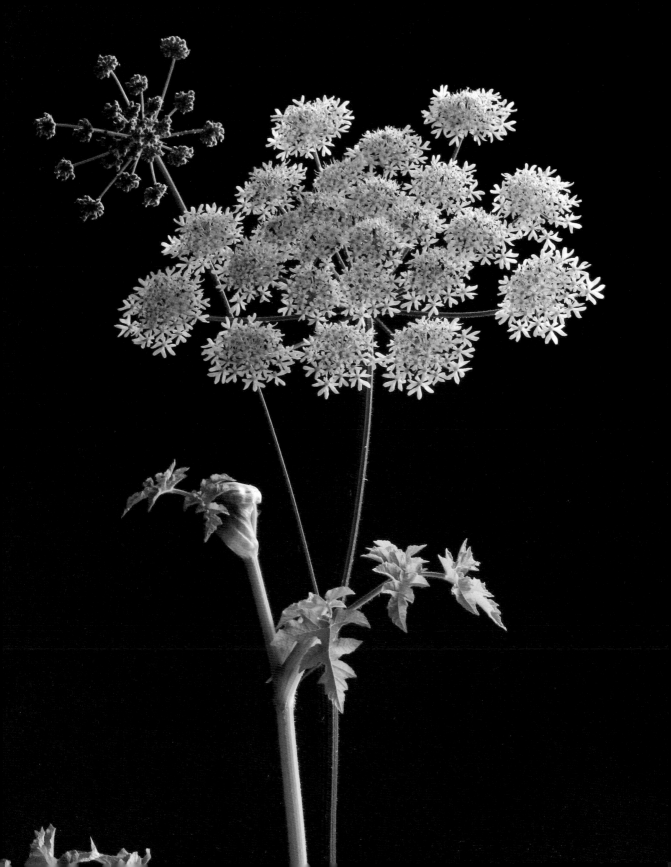

Below: hogweed flower bud packets in early summer. We call them knuckles: a succulent cooked treat.

Overall hogweed is a friendly wild flower / weed, a usually benevolent emblem of summer, while giant hogweed is more threatening, alien.

The principal issue is the sap, which is potentially phototoxic in hogweed but dangerously so in giant hogweed. When released by efforts to strim or cut down giant hogweed shoots, especially in hot, humid conditions, a watery exudate emerges that contains furanocoumarin glycosides.

These glycosides can photosensitize our skin to severe UV damage, with large, painful blisters appearing, to be followed by ulcers that heal to leave purplish or even black scars. Sap finding its way into the eyes can lead to problems, even blindness.

Another question: is hogweed really food for pigs? Certainly it was in the past, when people often kept a domestic pig.

Taking the other element of the name, is it a weed? It is in our garden, popping up everywhere, and it grows freely along road verges and field margins. We appreciate it as a beautiful structural plant that helps support other floppier garden plants.

The history of hogweed

Some 12,000 years ago, as the great icecaps retreated near the Bering Strait, ancestors of modern Native American peoples moved across the land bridge and south into an almost uninhabited continent.

Among the plants they found and consumed as they travelled was hogweed / cow parsnip. This has remained an important vegetable for Native Americans until today, with the masterly ethnobotanical survey by Nancy Turner (2014) recording cow parsnip in 45 native languages from the American northwest and interior.

Turner relates how on the west coast people would travel long distances in spring to favorite gathering places with the best-tasting cow parsnip plants. The shoots growing in shade were said to be milder-tasting and preferred to those in full sun.

Provision for winter was made by sun-drying the stems or preserving them in seal oil. Such information was passed down the generations.

Also from the far north, the original recipe for borsch soup in Siberia and Kamchatka featured lacto-fermented cow parsnip. It is only in the last

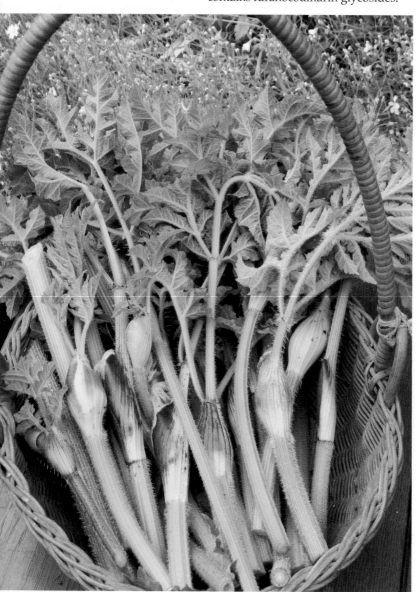

century or so that borscht has been considered to be beet-based.

The British science and botany writer Phoebe Lankester (1825–1900) noted how in the Siberia and Russia of her time hogweed stalks were dried out in the sun. The sweet sap that exuded from the stalks crystallized to give a summer delicacy. The stalks yielded a spirit when distilled with bilberries.

Like their Northern American counterparts, the Steppe dwellers boiled the stems and leaves of cow parsnip as a staple green vegetable.

Modern-day foragers have rediscovered this forgotten use of a familiar weed, with impetus given by writer/photographer Roger Phillips. His pioneering 1983 book *Wild Food* declared that hogweed shoots are *unequivocally one of the best vegetables I have eaten*. Many, including us, agree.

Herbal & other uses of hogweed

When children were allowed and even encouraged to roam free – within living memory of the postwar boomer generation – everybody knew hogweed was for making blow-pipes or pea-shooters. The plant was easy to identify, was found everywhere, and the stems were hollow and rigid yet still readily cuttable.

But who would have thought, as Nancy Turner relates from western North America, that the stalks were also good as snorkels when swimming underwater, or that hogweed roots made a good bear trap mixture?

Medicinally, the roots were boiled into a cow parsnip tea in the American colonies. This was drunk to ease colic, cramps, headaches, colds, flu and tuberculosis. Poultices using the plant were put on sores, bruises, stiff joints, warts and boils.

In European herbalism the great Swedish systematizer Linnaeus knew hogweed as a sedative in the mid-18th century. In his 1597 *Herball* John Gerard

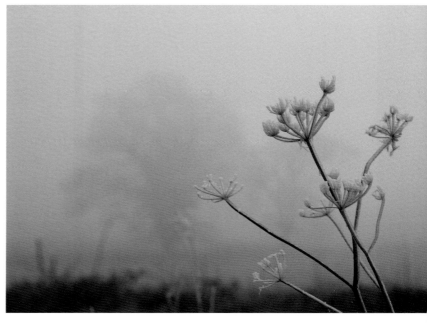

advised an oil of the leaves and roots for treating headache and lethargy. A century later, in 1707, John Pechey wrote that hogweed root is *Emollient and asswages Tumors*, while the *Seed is excellent for* [treating] *Hysterik Fits* [epilepsy].

The plant has been little used medicinally in recent centuries, but, interestingly, modern pharmaceutical research has explored older beliefs.

The *Heracleum* genus in general has experimentally demonstrated anti-asthmatic, memory and 'alertness-improving' effects. Hogweed has shown properties of reducing high blood pressure, while its essential oil can destroy certain human melanoma and carcinoma cells.

In terms of insect pollinators, a paper by Marcin Zych (2007) identified 107 species visiting hogweed flowers in Poland, including many flies, bumblebees, beetles and butterflies.

Paul Evans summed up well in a 2019 *Guardian* article, suggesting the Apiaceae are *far more important to insects*, and *saving the insects is the last great labor of Hercules* (a play on the genus name of hogweed).

Above: in winter remnants of hogweed make striking skeletal shapes in the garden and along roadsides

Below: fresh green and the smaller dried seeds of hogweed, about life-size

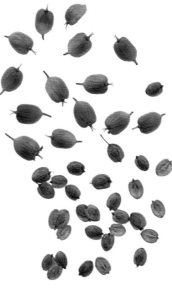

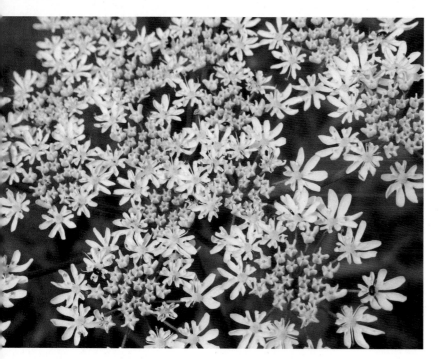

The dazzling patterns of
hogweed flowers

How to eat hogweed

The first rule in hogweed cooking,
as with any wild food, is to be 100%
certain of the identity of the plant.
The best way to learn is to walk with
a trusted forager and follow his/her
advice. You need to see, smell, touch
and get the 'jizz' (outline shape) of the
plant in its habitat to be totally certain
of what it is.

Botany field guides and videos are
next best in helping you specify that
your carrot species is indeed hogweed,
though phone apps are less reliable.

Be careful in collecting. People with
sensitive skins can react to the mildly
phototoxic elements in hogweed sap
and come out in blisters. Wear gloves
if in doubt, and avoid the sap on hot
sunny midsummer days when it is
most chemically active.

For both cow parsnip and hogweed,
custom and experience suggested that
once the flowers appear there is too
much build-up of bitter elements for
pleasant eating. This is learned wisdom
we can apply to our own experiments.

We count four seasons for hogweed
eating. First, young shoots in spring
are delightful when a few inches high.
Early picking may ensure a second
flush later on. These shoots are tasty
blanched for a few minutes, then oil
and condiments added. As with all
parts of the plant, making into soup is
an option. But our favorite way to eat
them is as tempura (p144).

A second season, and still more
spring than summer, sees the young
flower stalks coming through. Once
the structural ribs develop, peeling is
advisable as they can be quite bristly.
Cook as for the shoots. Some foragers
like this season best of all.

Third, in early summer, come the
young flower buds. Before opening,
the unfurled flowers are enclosed in
an unmistakable swollen, purplish
or diaphanous bundle several inches
across, known in our family as
'knuckles', and are a bit like broccoli.

We made a note on 21 May one year:
*two knuckles cooked this morning, sliced
and fried with mushrooms, with added
tamari. They were lovely, with a taste
between citrus and lovage. Not a meal for
every day but good as a treat or to titillate a
guest's taste buds.*

For different people, the flavor of
hogweed/cow parsnip can evoke
asparagus or celery, parsnip or lovage;
often mandarin or orange are cited
as back notes. The combined taste
experience has a characteristic intensity
that we think you will like.

The final season is the seeds, when the
citrus sensation strengthens. Eating
one or two seeds while they are still
green gives a pleasant, buzzy, head-
clearing sensation, but you may feel
light-headed if you eat more than two
or three. Be careful!

But once they turn brown and ripe,
the seeds are more mellow, less 'heady'.
We enjoy them as a flavor in biscuits
(cookies) (p145), and in a seed cake
(p146).

Creamy Hogatoni

Young flower stalks of hogweed are delicious peeled and cooked. They can be used like rigatoni, or cut into circles and fried. They also make good tempura.

Pick a **double handful of young hogweed stems**. Peel them and cut into short pieces. Cook briefly in **boiling water** until tender – about 2 minutes – then rinse under **cold water** to stop them cooking.

In a small saucepan, combine **2 tablespoons olive oil**, **2 cloves minced garlic** and **3 tablespoons oat cream**. Cook for a couple of minutes, then remove from heat and add **1 tablespoon yeast flakes**, and then the cooked hogweed stalks.

Toss to coat evenly. **Salt to taste**. Sprinkle with **grated vegan cheese** or **toasted almond flakes**. Serve immediately.

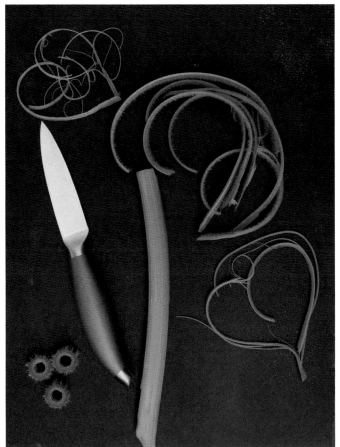

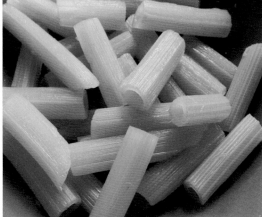

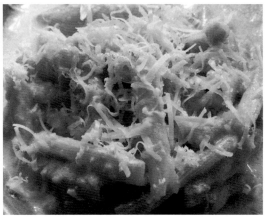

Hogweed **Paella**

Heat **1 tablespoon extra virgin olive oil** in a paella pan or large frying pan.

Cook over gentle heat: **1 onion, chopped** and **1 shallot, chopped**
When soft and beginning to brown, add **2 cloves garlic**, minced or finely sliced
After a minute or so, add **200g (1 cup) short grain brown rice**
Stir to coat the rice in the oil, then add **1 teaspoon smoked paprika, a pinch of saffron strands or turmeric powder** and **2 bay leaves**
Add **3 cups (700ml) hot vegetable stock**
Simmer for 30 minutes, stirring occasionally.

While the rice is cooking, grill **3 red peppers**, cut into thirds
When the skin is blistering or beginning to turn black, remove and let cool. Once cool, the skins should pull off easily. Slice the peeled peppers.

Blanch **a double handful of hogweed buds** in **boiling, salted water** for about a minute. Drain and rinse under cold water.

In a small frying pan, gently cook **1 tablespoon extra virgin olive oil** and **5 or 6 mushrooms, sliced**.

When the mushrooms are nearly done, add **½ cup pitted black olives** and the blanched hogweed buds. Cook for another couple of minutes.

When the rice has simmered for 30 minutes, add the sliced grilled red peppers and the mushroom, olive and hogweed mixture.

Optional extras:
a handful of pea pods or green beans
a cup of cooked chickpeas (garbanzos)

Cook for another 15 minutes, adding another **125ml (½ cup) or so of stock or water** if needed. If the rice is still chewy after 15 minutes, put a lid on the pot and cook for a few minutes longer.

Alternatives: Squeeze a little lemon juice over and sprinkle with chopped parsley or chopped nipplewort leaves just before serving.

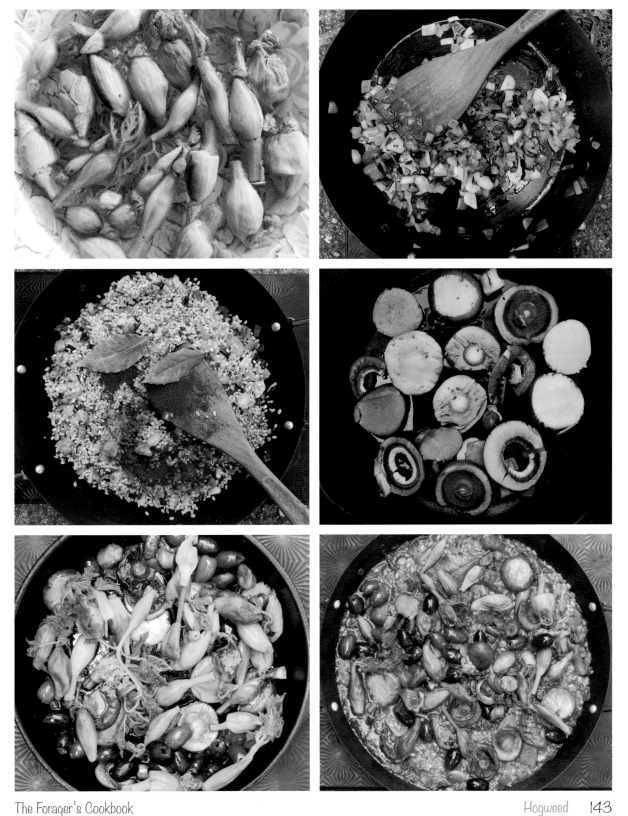

Hogweed Tempura

The young leaves of hogweed make wonderful tempura. Pick them when they are either still folded at the base of the plant, or when they open out but are still small. The young leaves first appear in the early spring, but especially if you keep picking them, they can also be found later in the year.

To make the batter, mix **120g (1 cup) flour** with **1 tablespoon cornflour (cornstarch)** and enough **cold water** to make a thin batter. Dip a young hogweed leaf into the batter to thinly coat it, shaking off any excess, then drop into **hot vegetable oil to deep fry** until light golden.

Put on a rack or on kitchen roll (paper towel) to drain, and serve while still hot with your favorite dipping sauce.

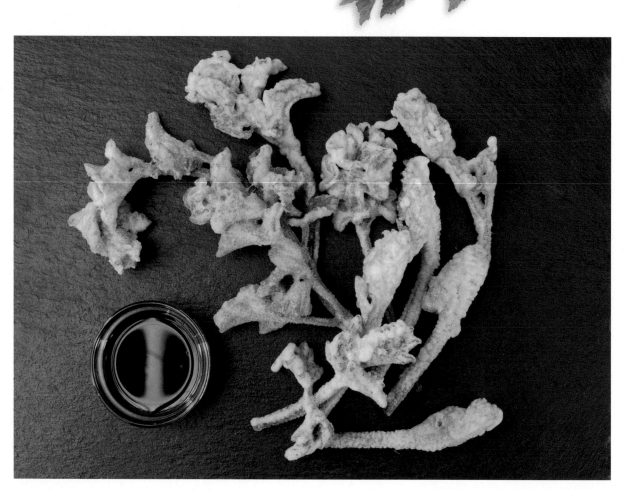

Hogweed Biscuits (Cookies)

Preheat your oven to 160C/325F.

Warm **170g (6oz) solid vegan butter**, **160g (¾ cup) golden granulated sugar** and **85g (¼ cup) golden syrup or maple syrup** in a small saucepan until just melted.

When melted, transfer to a bowl, then mix in **360g (3 cups) plain flour or spelt flour**, **2 teaspoons baking soda** and **1 tablespoon ground ripe hogweed seed**.

The mixture should come away cleanly from the sides of the bowl and make a ball.

Roll walnut-sized pieces in your hands and place on baking parchment on baking sheets, leaving room for them to spread. You can flatten them slightly with your hand.

Bake for about 10 minutes or until golden. The color turns quite quickly so keep an eye on them when they are nearly done. Cool on a wire rack.

Makes 30 to 40 biscuits (cookies).

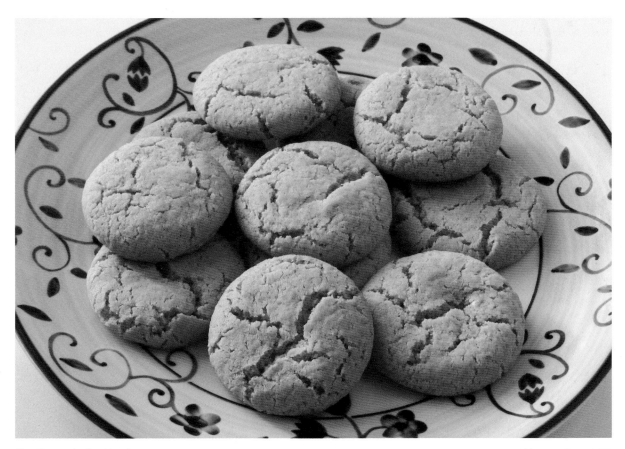

Hogweed Seed Cake

This is a firm cake, like a gingerbread but with the citrus tones of ripe hogweed seed. Other spices can be added, but it's also lovely with just hogweed. Preheat oven to 160C/325F.

Warm together in a bowl:
110 g (½ cup) maple syrup or 350g (1 cup) golden syrup (light treacle)
220g (1 cup) vegan butter, or 120ml (½ cup) coconut oil and 120ml (½ cup) sunflower oil
250ml (1 cup) water with **1 teaspoon baking soda (bicarbonate of soda)** dissolved in it

Mix together in another bowl:
480g (4 cups) flour
200g (1 cup) sugar
1 tablespoon hogweed seed powder
1½ teaspoons cinnamon

Stir both sets of ingredients together until well mixed. It should be quite a thick, smooth batter.

Pour into a greased tin, allowing room for it to rise. We use an oval tin 21 by 25cm (8 by 10in), with high sides, or a large and a small loaf tin. Bake in a moderate oven 160C/325F for 1 hour (if you are using loaf tins they will take less time – check after 40 minutes). The cake should be golden on top, and a straw poked into the center should come out clean.

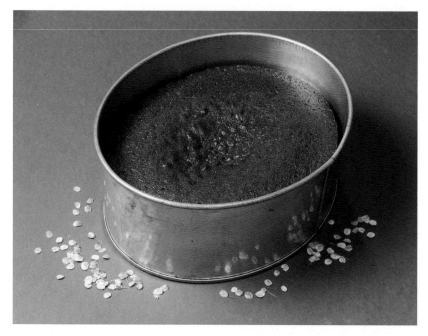

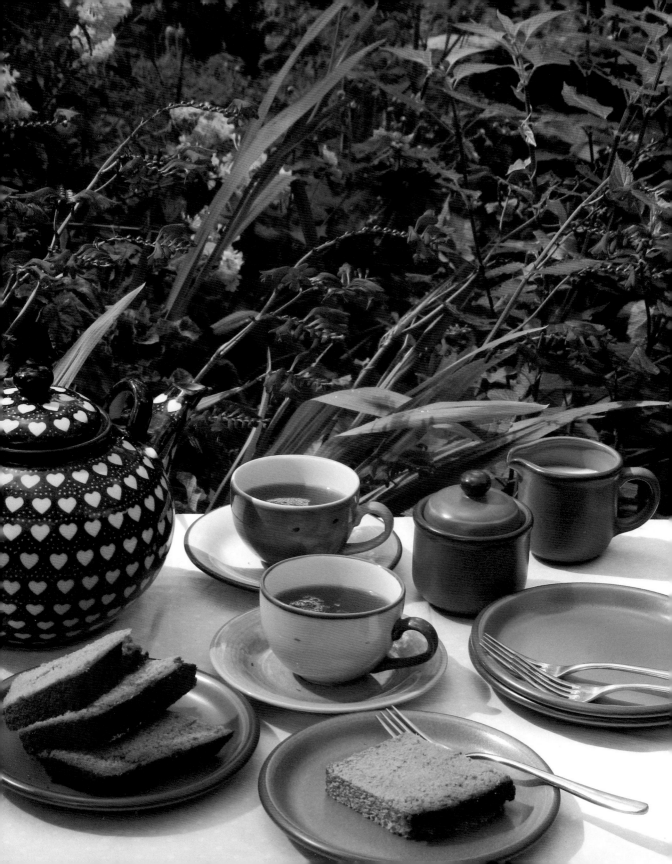

Honey Mushroom

Gardeners revile honey fungus or honey mushroom (*Armillaria mellea*), but it is the wild mushroom we both eat most. It tastes delicious, we are confident we can safely identify it, and it is abundant in our garden every autumn. We cook some fresh and dry plenty more to use throughout the year. An amazing colonizer, it has a strong mushroomy taste.

Basidomycetes
Armillaria mellea
Edible parts: young caps of fruiting bodies, fresh or dried

Distinguishing features: see text on right, **Identifying your honey mushroom**, especially small scales on the cap and a white spore print

There are at least seven closely related species of *Armillaria*.

Cautions: The main caution is to be absolutely certain of your identification, as with any wild mushroom. Some people suffer stomach upsets from eating honey mushroom. Do not eat raw.

Dangerous lookalikes:
The funeral bell, *Galerina marginata*, also grows in overlapping colonies, but is a darker color, has a smell that isn't mushroomy, and the **spore print is red-brown**. It is poisonous.

The sulphur tuft, *Hypholoma fasciculare*, abundant in Europe and North America, grows in clumps, is sulphur-color rather than honey, darkening to brown; stem often curved, with a darker cap center; yellow gills that go olive green; faint rings; **spore print purplish to black**, mushroomy smell. Inedible, bitter, poisonous.

What kind of a weed is honey mushroom?

We have chosen to use the American name of honey mushroom rather than honey fungus, because we deal more with the edible aspect (the fruiting body we can see) than the whole organism (the mycelium underground). It also sounds more appetizing.

Can we justify it as a weed? In our garden it certainly acts like one. It comes up in places we would rather it left alone, it grows rampant and it kills trees, especially exotic species (it did for our ten-year-old, 20-foot high paulownia and a ginkgo tree); it also hurried two silver birches, a lilac and an ornamental cherry to their ends, but admittedly they were old and tired.

What kind of a weed, then, are we dealing with? A hugely destructive root parasite in many forests and gardens, attacking both coniferous and broad-leaf trees and other plants. It is the number one weed problem on the leading British gardening website.

There are at least seven species of honey mushroom recognized. In Britain two of them (*Armillaria mellea*, and the less frequent *A. ostoyae*, dark honey fungus) thrive both on dead/decaying and live tree roots, while five other species depend on already dead trees.

The 'white rot' damage caused isn't easily quantified financially, with both actual losses and opportunity losses from unplanted trees involved. Reputationally, honey mushroom is a pariah. There are no easy preventive measures or methods of control. But you can eat them.

Its common names bootlaces or shoestrings (in the US) reference its rhizomorphs. These are its main method of spread, travelling a meter (3.3ft) underground in a year, or more in warmer and humid seasons.

Looking like old-fashioned black cassette tape, and nearly as difficult to cut, the rhizomorphs carry far more of the colony's distribution load than the spores. They spread along root paths between trees, such that in an ancient forest practically every tree might become affected.

Honey mushroom appears in summer or autumn and its fruiting cycle is rapid. In one recent year in our garden it appeared in October, lasted two weeks and then decayed, as it will, into a smelly black goo.

Identifying your honey mushroom

Before considering eating honey mushroom, though, please be certain of your ID. **Only eat something you are totally sure meets the following tests**:

1. honey mushroom forms colonies of overlapping clumps at the base of infected trees, tumbling like a favela on a hillside.

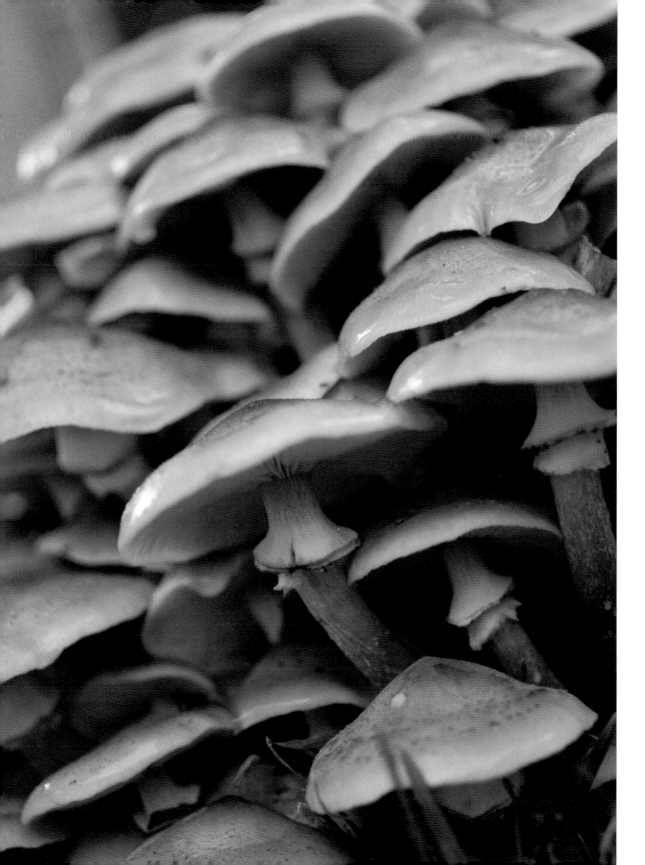

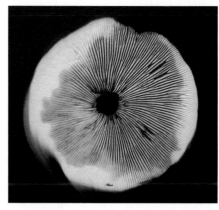

To make a spore print: cut off a recently opened honey mushroom cap, discard the stalk, turn the cap upside down on a dark-colored piece of paper. Leave overnight and check the spore print next day. Or, in the honey mushroom colony, visually examine the lower level, which may have white spores from specimens above, looking like the lightest touch of snow.

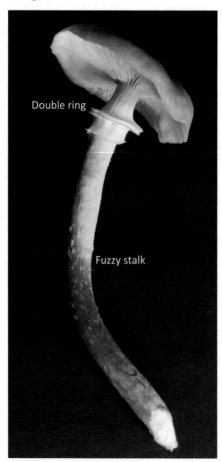

Double ring

Fuzzy stalk

2. specimens have an overall honey color with a darker brown center in the cap, with **tiny beard-stubble-like scales** (see photo on right) which may wash away in older specimens

3. gills are close-set, continuous with the stem (stipe), fused at the base, and white to creamy, turning yellowish

4. stem is whitish and later yellowish with a persistent single or double ring (skirt)

5. in maturity, stem is fuzzy below skirt

6. a pale **white spore print**

7. smell is variously described as mushroomy or spermatic, but is not strong.

So, most importantly, do not eat unless the small dark scales are present on the cap, and the spore print is white.

History and uses of honey mushroom

Returning to the honey mushroom as an organism, it is truly remarkable. It has been claimed as the largest single living being in the world and one of the oldest.

Merlin Sheldrake's wonderful book on fungi, *Entangled Life* (2020), tells of the current record holder in a mixed conifer forest in Oregon. This honey mushroom complex (*A. ostoyae*) weighs in at hundreds of tonnes, covers 10 sq. km (2,470 acres) and is anywhere from 2,000 to 8,000 years old.

A similarly huge forest colony in Michigan was found to have a very slow rate of genetic mutation, which perhaps protects it against damage to its DNA, a stability that Sheldrake suggests might enable its extreme age.

Honey mushroom is also a traditional medicinal, particularly in China. Recent pharmacological research has supported the use in anti-cancer applications of an aromatic ester, armillaridin, derived from the mushroom.

A tincture from the mycelium has been found, in studies on mice, to have potential in treating Alzheimer's disease.

Another area of action is for treating epilepsy, Parkinson's, vertigo and Ménière's disease. Julie has found dried honey mushroom decoction to be a specific treatment for postviral vertigo.

Research into the endangered Chinese medicinal orchid *Gastrodia elata*, the potato orchid, which is symbiotic with honey mushroom, shows that the mushroom duplicates the orchid's medicinal action.

The Chinese medicine Tian ma, made from Gastrodia root, is well known for treating headaches, dizziness and amnesia. If honey mushroom could be substituted for it, it would certainly have abundance, cheapness and sustainability on its side.

How to eat honey mushroom

Honey mushroom caps have a tender rather than a 'meaty' texture, so they combine well with other mushrooms. When dried, they have a strong 'mushroomy' aroma and flavor.

Honey mushroom wild-gathered in Russia is said to be appreciated even above morels and chanterelles. Honey mushroom pierogi dumplings are made in the Ukraine. A close relative, the rare matsutake or pine mushroom, is a delicacy in Japan.

The harvest season is short as the mushrooms need to be picked young (a few days). If you have a glut, drying some is a good idea – we use our dehydrator for this. Rehydration is quick and the flavor is noticeably enhanced. The stalks are rather too tough to eat, especially when dried. Do not eat the mushrooms raw.

If you haven't eaten honey mushroom before, try a small amount to start with in case of any adverse reaction.

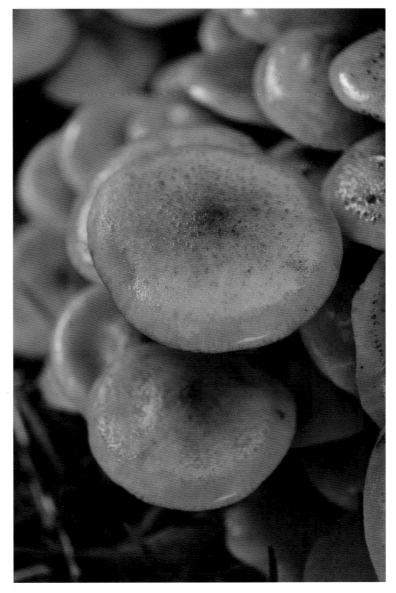

Some people like to boil their honey mushrooms and discard the water before frying them, but we haven't found it necessary, nor that eating the mushroom gave us tummy wobbles except for one time when we left them sitting unused until the following day before cooking.

So please gather and cook them or dry them as soon as possible afterwards – don't leave them hanging around.

Honey mushrooms usually appear in wet weather in the autumn. The darker brown center of the cap and the small, rough beard-stubble-like scales are key identifying features.

Honey Mushroom

Honey Mushroom Glazed Peppers

Tear about **20g (2 cups) dried honey mushrooms** into small pieces, discarding the stems. Put them in a bowl and pour on **1 cup boiling water**. Leave for about 15 minutes to rehydrate.

Meanwhile, sauté **150g (1 cup) finely diced onion** in **1 tablespoon oil**. When the onions are becoming transparent, add about **100g (3½ oz) sliced mixed fresh mushrooms** and **3 or 4 cloves of minced garlic**. Cook a couple of minutes, then add the honey mushrooms, removed from their soaking water (they will have absorbed most of it). Continue cooking for 5 or 10 minutes. Add **½ teaspoon rubbed sage** and **1 teaspoon fennel seeds**.

Put **75g (½ cup) dried breadcrumbs** in a small bowl, and add about **5 tablespoons hot water** to moisten them – the exact amount you need will depend on the breadcrumbs. Mix with the mushroom mixture. Add the **finely grated zest of a lemon**.

Toast **100g (¾ cup) whole hazelnuts**, either in a dry pan or in the oven until just turning golden. Cool, then rub off the skins. Crush by pressing with the side of a big knife blade. (An electric grinder tends to give a fine powder and a few big chunks.)

Mix up to half the crushed hazelnuts into the mushroom mixture, and reserve the rest to go on top of the stuffed peppers.

Cut **4 Romano peppers** in half lengthwise, and remove the seeds. Fill with the stuffing, and arrange in a baking dish. Top with the remaining hazelnuts.

Bake at 175C/350F for 20 minutes.

While they are baking, make a balsamic glaze by putting **125ml (½ cup) balsamic vinegar**, **½ teaspoon cornflour (cornstarch)** and **1 tablespoon maple syrup** in a small saucepan. Bring to the boil, and stir for a minute or two just until it becomes clear. It will thicken as it cools.

Sprinkle the baked peppers with chopped parsley or nipplewort, and drizzle about a tablespoon of the balsamic glaze on each.

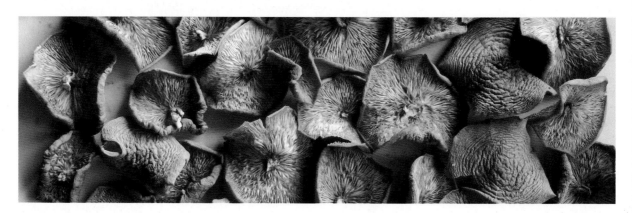

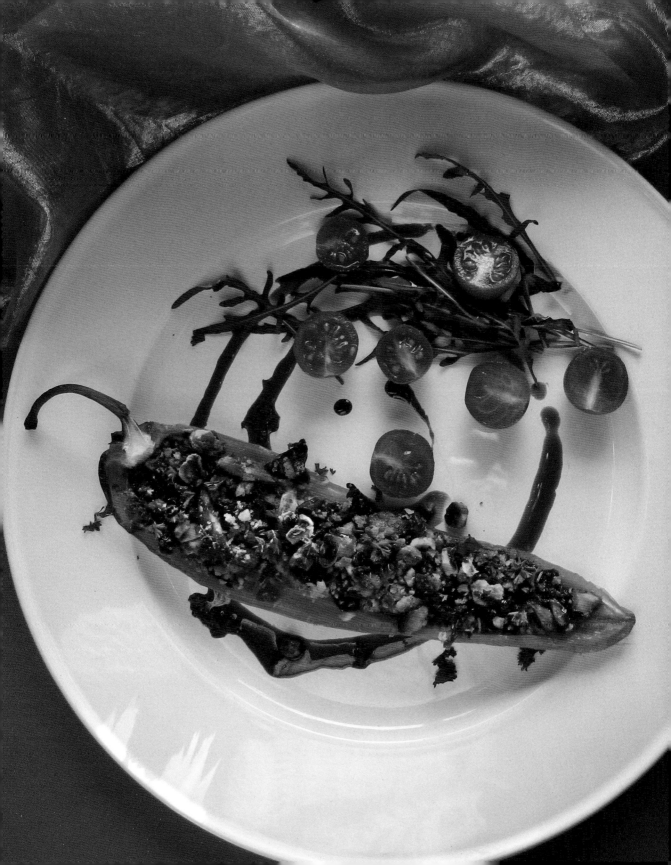

Honey Mushroom with **Paprika**

This recipe is loosely inspired by Hungarian paprika and goulash recipes. We make this with fresh honey mushrooms, or dried ones briefly soaked in hot water and mixed with other kinds of fresh mushrooms. This amount serves two.

Finely dice **an onion**. Fry in **a little oil** until translucent. Add **1 or 2 cloves garlic, minced**, and **225g (3 cups) sliced honey mushrooms** and cook for about 5 minutes.
Add **1 tablespoon sweet or smoked paprika**, and **170ml (¾ cup) coconut milk**.
Add **salt to taste**. Simmer gently for about 10 minutes, adding more coconut milk or some water if it becomes dry.

Serve over rice or flat noodles.

Alternatives: You can add red peppers with the mushrooms and chopped tomatoes with the coconut milk.
If you like spicy food, add some hot paprika or a little chilli powder. Cashew or oat cream can be used instead of the coconut milk.
If you are using dried honey mushrooms, use about a cupful, soaked in hot water for 5 minutes, and 2 cups of fresh mushrooms. The texture of chestnut mushrooms or maitake combine well with the more delicate honey mushrooms.

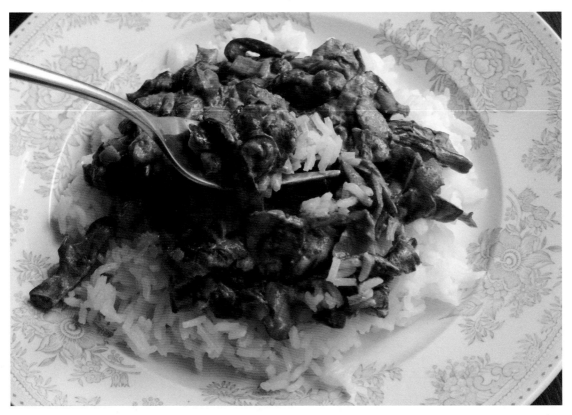

Honey Mushroom **Risotto**

Heat some oil in a saucepan. Add **a mugful of arborio or other risotto rice** (about 250g), **1 shallot or small onion**, finely diced, and **a handful of sliced fresh mushrooms** – these can be wild mushrooms, chestnut mushrooms or ordinary button mushrooms. Cook gently for about 5 minutes.

Add **½ cup dried honey mushroom pieces**. Remove the stems and tear caps into pieces. You don't need to soak them for this recipe, as the broth will rehydrate them quickly.

You'll need about **3 mugfuls hot vegetable stock**. Add the stock slowly, a ladleful at a time, allowing each ladleful to be absorbed before adding the next, stirring as you go. Keep going until the rice is plump and just tender. You may not need all the stock – you don't want the rice to become mushy.

Salt to taste. Stir in ¼ **cup yeast flakes (nutritional yeast)** just before serving. If you like, sprinkle each serving with a little chopped parsley, chives or wild garlic.

Alternatives: When we were in Anghiari, northern Italy, a few years ago we had a most wonderful *fruits of the forest* risotto, which had mushrooms with dried blackcurrants and raspberries, then truffle shavings served on top. The dried berries give the creamy risotto a refreshing tang. You could also finish the risotto off with chopped toasted hazelnuts.

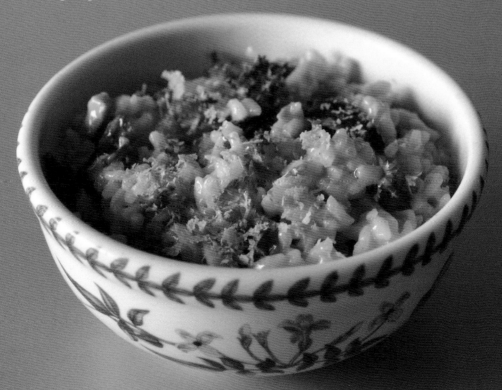

Jack by the Hedge

Jack by the hedge (*Alliaria petiolata*) is also called garlic mustard because it tastes of both flavors. It is a common hedgerow, wayside and garden plant, preferring damp and shady places. We like to eat it with mash, in wraps, as sushi and in stir fries.

**Brassicaceae
(formerly Cruciferae)
Cabbage family**

Biennial.

Distinguishing features:
Handsome, upright spring plant, growing along field and wood edges, hedgebanks, riversides and gardens. Flowers in late spring at up to 1m (3.3ft) tall. The flowers are small, with four snowy white petals, contrasting with the bright green lush foliage of crinkly, heart-shaped leaves; seed pods are thin, held at an angle to the stalks.

When and what to harvest:
The whole plant is edible. Pick young leaves in spring, flower buds in spring, flowers in late spring and roots in autumn & winter.

Sulphoraphane ... can cross the blood–brain barrier and actually reverse damage caused by free radicals, and even normal aging.
– Sherzai & Sherzai (2021)

The flavor is bitter at first, but the warm, garlicky flavor that follows wins over most people.
– Irving (2009)

What kind of a weed is Jack by the hedge?

We prefer 'Jack by the hedge' to the more prosaic name 'garlic mustard', which is accurate for the taste spectrum of this cabbage species but often leads to confusion with the equally abundant hedge mustard (*Sisymbrium officinale*).

A West Country name for it is 'sauce alone', and Culpeper (1652) uses this as his main name. The foraged leaves were indeed boiled into a spring sauce, with 'alone' referring to 'ail', the French word for garlic. The plant was and still can be the basis of a sauce that stands midway between garlic and mustard.

Old English names reflect Jack by the hedge's role as a standby, a famine food if needed. In Leicestershire it was beggarman's oatmeal, and in nearby Lincolnshire poor man's mustard; elsewhere it was penny hedge.

This information was choreographed by Geoffrey Grigson in his wonderful *The Englishman's Flora* (1958). He recognizes the beauty of the plant, and with his poet's eye notes its military posture: *In brilliant sunshine, in May, one is always freshly struck by platoons of this familiar plant, at starched attention, the starch-white flowers above the new green leaves and against the green bank.*

But try telling this to foresters in the eastern US, where Jack by the hedge, introduced in 1868, is an unwanted invasive, with no natural predators, is self-fertilizing and produces chemicals that inhibit other plants and mycorrhizal fungi needed for tree seedling survival.

Jack by the hedge poses a threat not only to American native trilliums, spring beauty and wild ginger, but also to the forest itself. What is a relatively easily controlled weed in its native Europe has become a noxious (notifiable) menace in over thirty US states.

The history of Jack by the hedge

In 2013 the archaeologist Hayley Saul and colleagues published a study of charred food remains found on beaker pottery in Denmark and Germany some 6,000 years old. Traces of Jack by the hedge in the pots were interpreted as evidence of its use as a food spice.

They suggest this is the oldest record of the spicing of food in European prehistoric culture, which *challenges the view that plants were exploited by hunter-gatherers and early agriculturalists solely for energy requirements, rather than taste.*

Isn't it heartening to think of our ancestors foraging Jack by the hedge close by a woodland, nibbling it and adding it to their food, savoring its taste as we can?

William Turner's *A New Herball* (1562) seems to have the first English

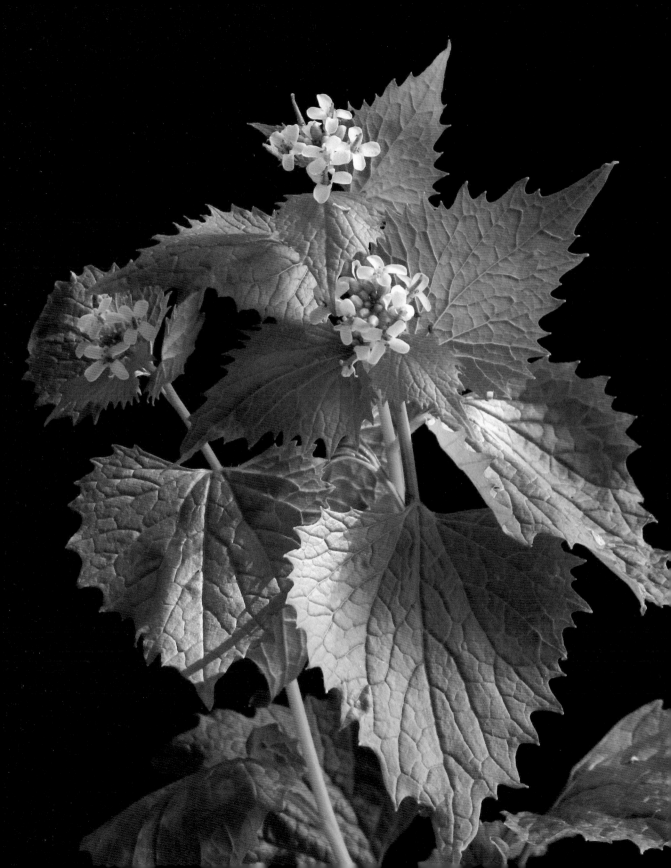

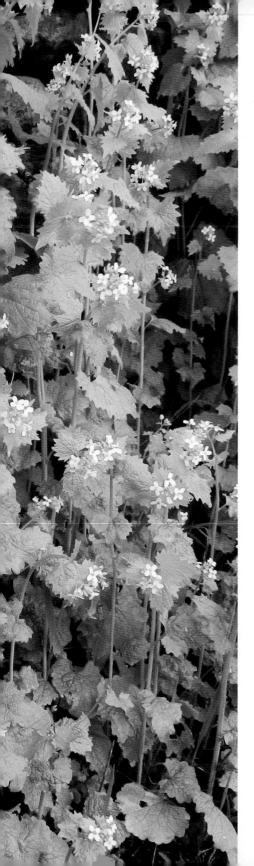

reference. He describes Jack by the hedge cooked as a spring sauce. Like other Brassicas – the mustards, cresses and pepperworts – it was relished as a condiment and boiled as a vegetable or added to a salad.

Today in our garden Jack by the hedge pops up as a weed among our flowers and vegetables, and we choose to welcome it as an upstanding and handsome wild plant favoring us with its company. It is a bonus that it is good to eat and to use herbally.

Herbal & other uses of Jack by the hedge

Gabrielle Hatfield (2007) notes that Jack by the hedge once had a role in 'official', or sanctioned medicine, when this was primarily plant-based. Until 1838, when *The British Herbal* ceased to list it, Jack by the hedge was a minor but useful treatment to induce sweating and was used externally as an antiseptic.

It also had a respected use in treating ulcers and gangrene. The esteemed Dutch doctor Herman Boerhaave posthumously published (1741) an account of boiling the leaves in wine and applying them to sores on a patient's leg that had become gangrenous following a neglected fracture.

Internally, leaves of Jack by the hedge boiled with honey or wine as a thick syrup were used to expectorate phlegm and treat coughs or hoarseness. The same preparations, or the leaves boiled as a decoction, made a hot drink to relieve the pain of edema (or dropsy, its old name), and asthma.

In addition to causing sweating, the leaves were said to be warming to the stomach and to aid digestion. Roots of a related wild Brassica, horseradish, are of course the ultimate in digestive 'warming'. The roots and seeds of Jack by the hedge were used similarly, but in lesser quantity than the leaves.

The Brassica family, including Jack by the hedge, has in recent times been researched as an exciting source of organosulphur compounds. One of these, sulforaphane, is said to be one of the most potent anti-cancer nutrients ever studied, and is important for brain health.

How to eat Jack by the hedge

All parts of the plant are edible, but the flower buds and young leaves are most often eaten. The flower buds can be cooked like broccoli, but retain a mustardy tang. The young tender flower stalks are sweet and make a tasty snack, or can be cooked like asparagus.

The leaves, at their best when young, combine well with mild creamy ingredients, either raw or cooked. Our recipes use them in mashed potato, wraps, sushi and stir fry. Another tasty option is rolling cooked risotto rice into two overlapping leaves to make a version of dolmades.

A new crop of leaves will often appear in autumn in areas with mild winters. These overwintering leaves are stronger in flavor than the young spring leaves, but are a welcome addition to winter recipes.

The thick white root can be grated like horseradish, to give a mustardy bite. It needs to be dug before the plant sends up a flowering stalk, after which it becomes woody.

Jack Mash

If your potatoes are young, there's no need to peel them.

Boil **1kg (2.2 lbs) potatoes** until tender. Drain, keeping some of the **cooking water**.

Put a thin layer of the cooking water back in the pan, and add
½ cup chopped Jack by the hedge
Cook for about a minute, just to wilt the leaves.

Add the potato back into the pan and mash.

Add **oat milk** – the amount will depend how dry and floury your potatoes are and how firm you like your mash.

Add **salt**, **pepper** and **oil** to taste.

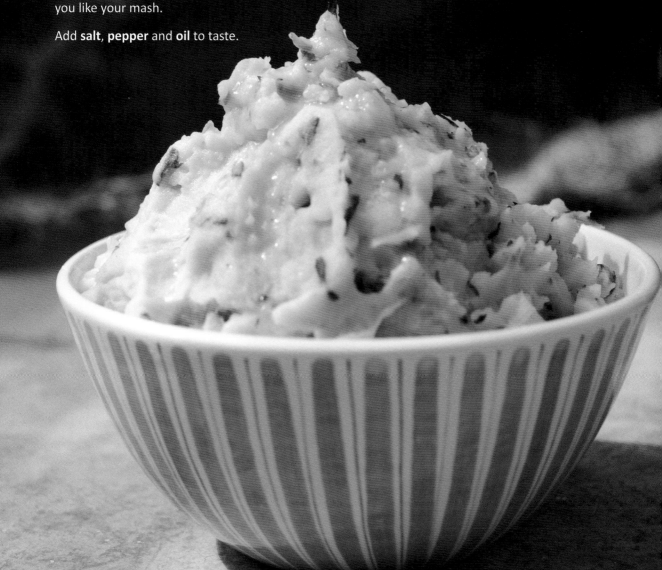

Jack **Wraps**

The mustardy flavor of Jack by the hedge goes really well in wraps. It combines well with creamy spreads, such as the cashew cream we use here. The raw cashews are ideally soaked in warm water for an hour or overnight, then drained, to make a smoother cream. But if you haven't got time, it also works with unsoaked nuts.

Blend **130g (1 cup) raw cashew nuts** with **1 tsp miso** and **enough water** to make the mixture into a smooth cream. Spread on **a wrap or tortilla**.

Arrange **young Jack by the hedge leaves** on top of the cashew cream, then arrange **sliced tomato** on top. Sprinkle with **salt** and **freshly ground black pepper** to taste.

Alternatives: Use hummus or mashed avocado as a spread instead of cashew cream. Try the chickweed hummus on p46. Cresses have a similar flavor and can be used instead of or in addition to the Jack by the hedge.

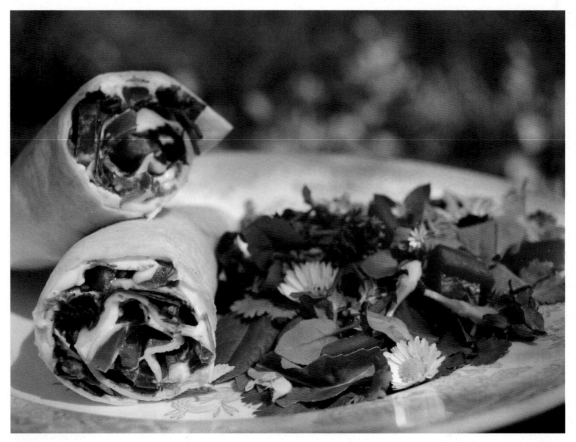

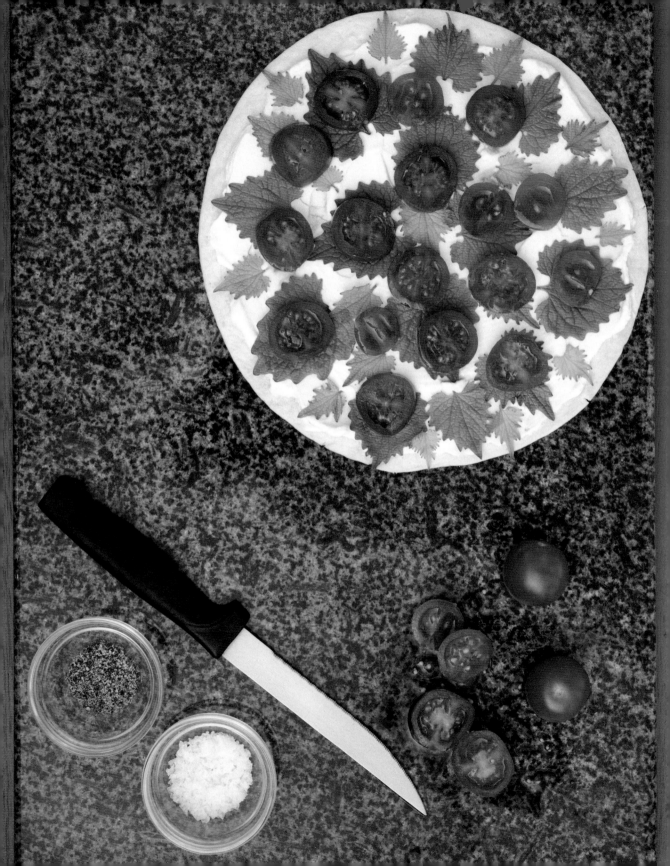

Jack Sushi

The peppery flavor of Jack by the hedge leaves combines well with the bland rice of sushi. If you haven't got a sushi mat, use a clean cloth to help you roll up the sushi.

Cook **200g (1 cup) sticky rice** with **½ teaspoon salt** and about **400ml water** in a covered saucepan, until all the water has been absorbed, then let sit. Or cook the rice according to the package instructions.

Stir in **½ tsp sugar** and **½ tsp rice wine vinegar or herbal vinegar**.
Taste, and add more if you want.

On a sushi mat, lay **2 sheets sushi nori**, then spread the cooked rice over the seaweed, leaving one edge uncovered. Lay your fillings somewhere near the middle of the rice. We used **1 or 2 carrots**, cut into thin ribbons with a peeler or mandoline, topped with **a handful of Jack by the hedge leaves**, cut into strips if large.

Roll up tightly, taking care not to roll the mat or cloth into your sushi. Cut with a very sharp knife.

The flavor develops more if left for a few hours or overnight, but they can be eaten straight away. Serve with a dipping sauce, such as the one on p206.

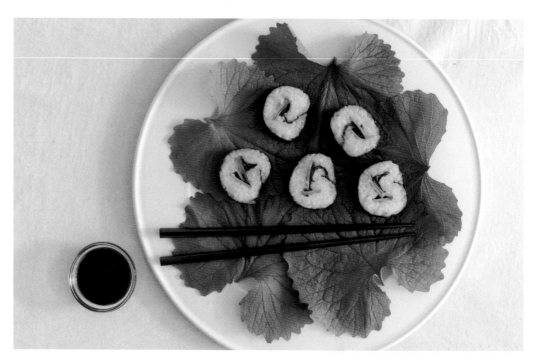

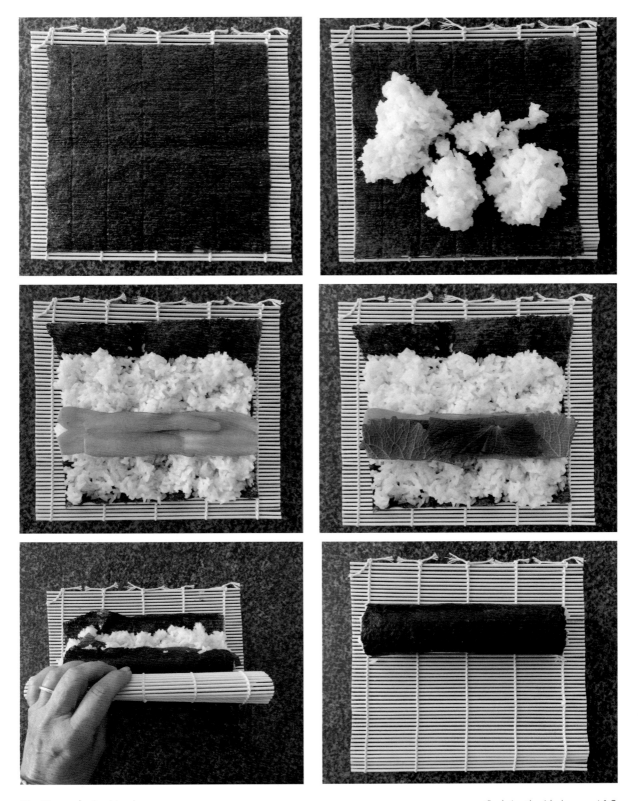

Jack Stir Fry

Prepare roughly **equal amounts of sliced red onion, coarsely grated carrot** and **Jack by the hedge budding tops or leaves**.

Heat **a little oil** in a wok, stir frying the onion for a minute or two. Then add the carrot, and stir fry for another minute or two. Add the Jack by the hedge budding tops and cook until wilted and bright green.

Season to taste with **soy sauce** and **toasted sesame oil**. Serve with **rice** or **noodles**.

Optional additions:
Add finely grated ginger
Add minced garlic
Add toasted sesame seeds

Alternatives: Cleavers tips, just before they flower, are also very good cooked this way.

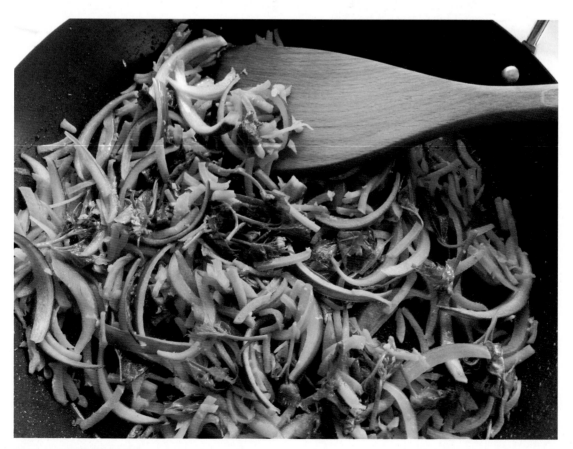

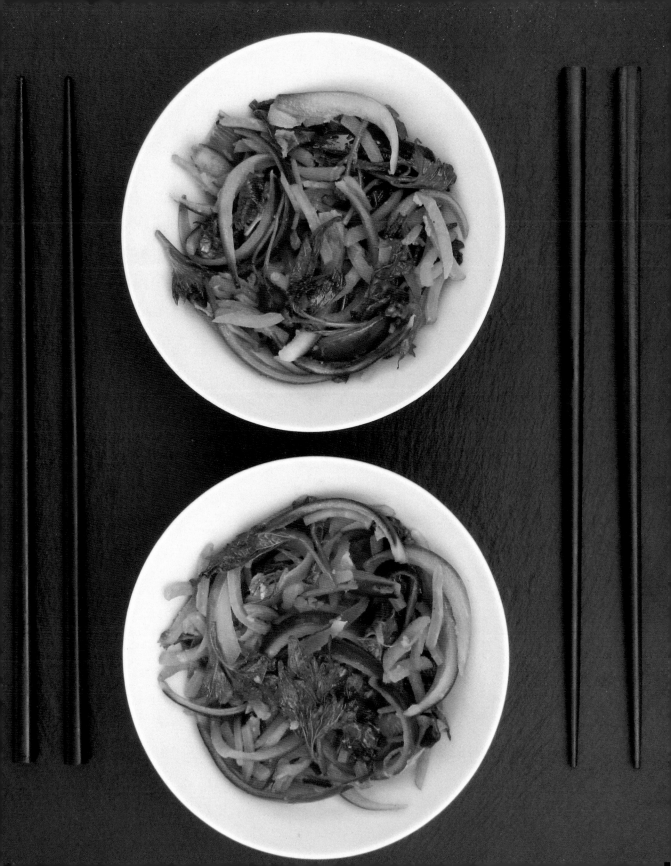

Mugwort

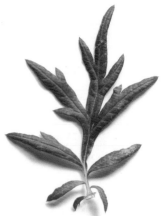

Mugwort is *Artemisia vulgaris*, which can be loosely interpreted as 'the gift from the goddess of healing to the people'. Now viewed as a weed, it was traditionally a 'female herb' but also long used for lucid dreaming and as moxa in acupuncture. Commercially important in food (e.g. tarragon) and drink (e.g. absinthe), we have found it is also excellent in rice, for soups and as a kefir.

**Asteraceae
(formerly Compositae)
Daisy family**

Perennial.

Edible parts: Flowering tops and leaves.

Distinguishing features: Statuesque and structural wild plant, up to 2m (6ft 6in) high, downy and somewhat aromatic. It has stout stems, often striped with purple, and wide-spreading side branches. Leaves are dark green on top, and covered in fine downy silver hairs beneath. The flowers are small and easily overlooked, with reddish-brown and yellow centers, emerging from silvery buds.

Related edible species: Japanese or Korean mugwort (yomogi), *Artemisia princeps*; tarragon, *A. dracunculus*; California mugwort, *A. douglasiana*, and many others worldwide.

Caution: Avoid excessive amounts of mugwort in pregnancy.

What kind of weed is mugwort?

Mugwort was not a plant Matthew knew as a youth. Perhaps it wasn't present in his neighborhood, but more likely it was there and he or his botanizing parents just didn't 'see' it.

More than most common plants (*vulgaris* in its name means abundant, as well as 'of the people'), mugwort merges into its background, even though it is tall and stately.

Its dark green leaves are somehow a neutral, unshowy background color, yet the silver effect of the under-leaves and the statuesque flower spike are handsome and pleasing.

Pattern recognition is involved here – making a form familiar enough to take on what birders call its 'jizz', its overall shape and character. Once somebody shows you mugwort – the personal touch beats using a book or app – you 'get' it and see it everywhere.

An irony arises: mugwort, not always seen, is a plant famed as promoting lucid dreaming, intense seeing.

But is it a weed, a nuisance, growing where not wanted? It flourishes and is appreciated in our own garden. In the wider world of weeds, it is a formidable player, surviving over most of the temperate world, often in frozen, dry or semi-arid areas.

First, it is hard to cut down, its fibrous stems resisting chopping (this also means the stems are too tough to eat); it is hard to pull out of the ground, with its dense root network frustrating gardeners and farmers alike.

Then it will grow back from the smallest piece of root left in the soil. These remnants act as root cuttings, giving evolutionary advantage to the many weeds that adopt this process. Shoots and leaves of mugwort have been regrown from remnants in the laboratory as well as roots.

Further, mugwort is allelopathic, meaning its roots emit a growth inhibitor that suppresses competing plants, whether other weeds or crops.

Mugwort is perennial and hardy – it has to be to thrive in the tundra and northern Japan. Its seeds are wind-distributed, but its main means of persistence are its thick rhizomes.

In *Artemisia* as a genus, there are about 400 species worldwide, including 170 from China, 55 from Europe and 50 from North America (Mabberley 2008).

One species, sweet annie (*A. annua*), yields high-quality artemisinin, a lactone used in malarial treatments.

The American sagebrushes are *Artemisias* rather than *Salvias* (sages). Best-known is big sagebrush

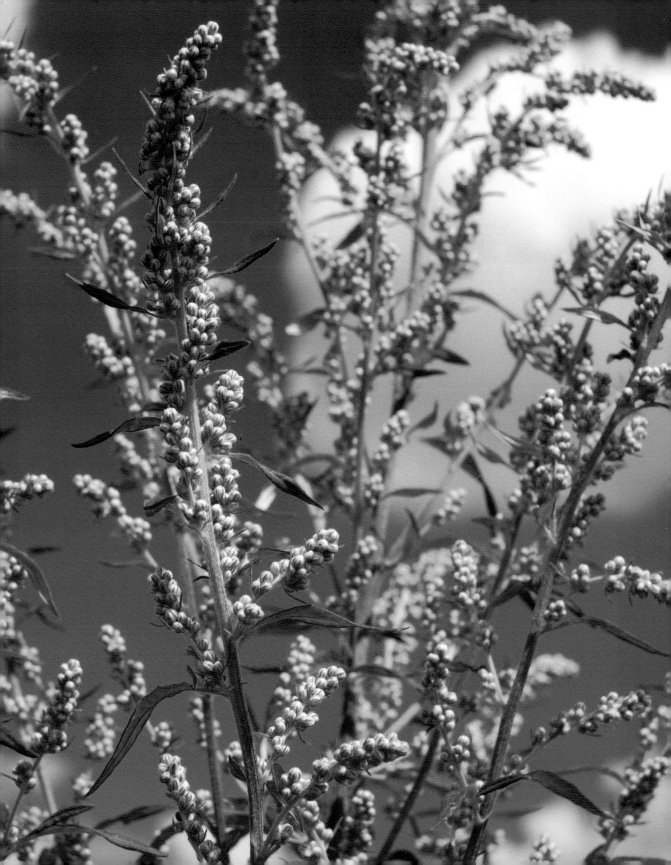

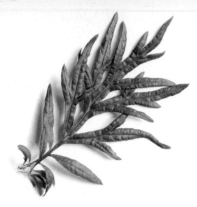

(*A. tridentata*), an abundant aromatic herb of the semi-arid mountain west.

There are native mugworts and sagebrushes in North America but also a number of introduced European species, which often compete for dominance in the same habitat.

The history of mugwort

Mugwort pollen is a strong presence in the glacial record over the last million years, though as the pollen is wind-distributed and may be carried far from source plants, its actual ancient on-the-ground presence is hard to ascertain.

It is cold weather-hardy, as shown in the 2006 discovery of *A. frigida* remains in the stomachs of mice preserved in the permafrost of the Yukon, Canada.

Given mugwort's formidable survival adaptations, it was probably abundant in the tundra and steppe grasslands crossed by wandering hunter-gatherers in post-glacial times. If they could 'see' it, they would have used it, especially for its smoke and as medicine.

In the historic record, mugwort is first noted in China and Japan some 2,500 years ago, as medicine and food. In China *A. argyri* was made into a green dumpling, known as *qingtuan*, with glutinous rice and aduki bean paste.

Qingtuan remains a spring delicacy, made commercially for the Qinming or tomb-sweeping (ancestor memorial) festival in April. Japan and Korea have similar old recipes for their local mugwort species.

In Europe, both Greek and Roman sources state that mugwort is already of venerable age and value. Greek myth calls it the first herb to be used by man, and mother's herb is an old Roman name.

In the first century AD, Pliny wrote that the name *Artemisia* was given in honor of Artemisia, queen of Caria, who knew the plant's virtues and taught them to women. This is perhaps the oldest reference to

mugwort as a specific herb for female use, equally at conception, childbirth and menstruation.

Almost a millennium later, the Anglo-Saxon leechbook of medical recipes credited the plant's name to the goddess Artemis, who ruled over the wilderness and the hunt, as well as medicine.

The leechbook said it was the centaur Chiron who gave herbal knowledge to Artemis, as indeed he did to Achilles (in respect of yarrow or *Achillea*).

Here mugwort is 'the eldest of worts', one of the nine sacred herbs of the Anglo-Saxons, and held to account for its ancient promise to help humanity.

By medieval times the pagan Artemis (or Diana) was supplanted by Christian exemplars, and St John's eve, 23 June, became the day mugwort was most celebrated, as a protector of man and beast alike in the coming summer.

In both Chinese and Western sources using mugwort strengthens you against the evil eye, demons, malignant gods, witchcraft and disease.

Herbal & other uses of mugwort

In modern times we lack the same faith in a plant's tutelary power, and prioritize its role in food and drink.

As food, the best-known species is tarragon (*A. dracunculus*). As drink, wormwood (*A. absinthum*) is the main ingredient of the once-banned liquor absinthe (with sweet fennel and anise); it also flavors the fortified wine vermouth. Black wormwood (*A. genipi*) is the basis of chartreuse and genepi.

Mugwort itself has been widely used in brewing ale, and some people believe its name means 'measure of the brew'. We use dried leaves in a kefir recipe.

The leaves make a refreshing tea, drunk hot or cold, and some modern-day foragers make a tasty mugwort mead; John Rentsen (2016) has blended it with ox-eye daisy to enjoyable effect.

[Artemisia afra is] one of the oldest and best-known of all the indigenous medicines in southern Africa, and has such diverse and multiple uses that it should be considered a significant tonic in its own right.
– Van Wyk & Gericke (2000)

If a footman take Mugwort and put it in his shoes in the morning he may goe forty miles before noon and not be weary.
– Coles (1656)

If they wad drink nettles in March / and eat muggins in May,/ Sae many braw maidens /wadna go to clay [die and be buried].
– traditional Scottish verse, Milliken & Bridgewater (2013)

Mugwort is an important herbal bitter for stimulating the liver and the digestion. It does not have the intensity of the related wormwood ('as bitter as wormwood' is an Old Testament simile) but has more herbal versatility.

A cup of mugwort tea or a glass of mugwort ale are good both before and after food, and mugwort's digestive profile also encompasses assisting patients with anorexia.

Mugwort can help regulate the flow of bile and break up fats. This explains its old use as a flavoring for cooked fatty meats like goose and pork, or oily fish. Equally, mugwort tea is useful when recovering from a rich meal and for treating indigestion or colic.

Spring leaves of mugwort were once a tonic for colds, coughs and sore throats; we have found these young leaves also make a good chewing gum. The smoke was often used an inhalant for headaches and congestion.

External medicinal uses of mugwort tea in some cultures included on a poultice for swellings, bruises, sores and, in North America, broken bones. The tea would be drunk at the same time.

But take note to avoid excessive mugwort in pregnancy. It contains small but appreciable amounts of thujones (the word is from *Thuja occidentalis*, the western red cedar).

Thujones are potentially implicated in spontaneous abortion, although the amount needed would be far more than in any course of mugwort herbal treatment.

The presence of thujones may lie behind mugwort's capacity to induce lucid dreaming. In Korea people respected the power of mugwort sufficiently to pluck the leaves only through a silk sleeve and not direct.

The plant is currently being researched for anti-tumor potential, and we have noted that sweet annie is grown as a commercial antimalarial.

In North America, many First Nations peoples relied on mugwort or sagebrush for fuel, tinder, cordage, fiber, clothing and roofing material. These uses can be emulated by crafts people and survivalists today.

We look at the varied uses of mugwort smoke on the next page ('Holy smoke').

Several species of mugwort, including southernwood (*A. abrotanum*) go into essential oils.

If we had just one word to describe mugwort it would be protection. This includes places as well as people.

We experienced this for ourselves a few years ago. A patient and later friend of Julie's has a small farm in south Norfolk, a couple of fields with a few cows. But what makes the farm extraordinary is that its earth has never been ploughed, as far as anyone knows, and no fertilizers or pesticides have ever contaminated it.

We had tears as we walked on this 'unimproved' land: the whole of England was once like this, Julie mused: organic, humming with insects, rich in birds and plants.

But the modern world of agrifarming was not far away. All around our friend's few acres are large, de-fenced fields of grain, produced with a full complement of chemicals. And the farmers have their eye on our friend's property – evil spirits indeed.

But between the two worlds, not planted but just appearing at the field edge, is a line of mugwort plants. They know their job.

How to eat mugwort
Essentially, dried mugwort leaves make an aromatic flavoring, adding stimulating bitterness to bland rice, beans or tofu. Mugwort has a capacity to intensify latent flavors, and a little crumble of leaves enhances even the most prosaic mushroom soup.

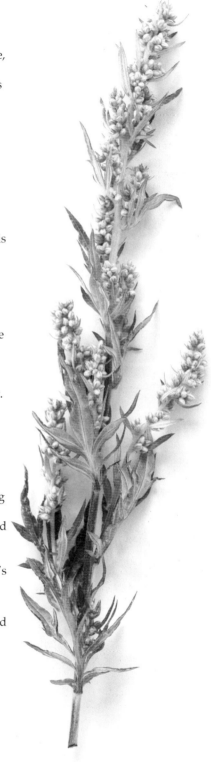

Holy smoke: mugwort magic

We began cooking experimentally with mugwort's aromatic smoke after seeing smoke-infusing on a TV cooking show. Our mugwort-flavored tofu features in a kebab recipe on p172.

Mugwort literally is 'a smoke'. Its rolled-up leaves were used before tobacco crossed the Atlantic to Europe, and within memory in parts of England a mugwort cigarette was a familiar young person's free introduction to adult intoxications. It was also known, disparagingly, as gypsy's tobacco or sailor's tobacco.

Powdered mugwort leaves became snuff in southern Africa (*Artemesia afra*), and in North America were an analgesic to relieve headaches or clear congestion. American cousins of mugwort, the sagebrushes, were smoked in First Nations pipes of peace in communal gatherings or in the aftermath of war. The fumes are restful and calming, especially in smudge sticks. In *Backyard Medicine* we relate how our smudging cleared the air during a teenage party. Mugwort is used as an aromatic cleansing smoke for sweat lodges, and in the Pacific northwest was a decontaminant of polluted areas.

A traditional use of mugwort smoke in China is as moxa, a technique of acupuncture. Moxa is prepared from *Artemesia argyri* or *A. vulgaris*, with the leaves dried, crushed and the remnant fibers made into small cones. The cones are then burnt on the top of the acupuncture needles or direct on the skin at the desired acupuncture point on a body meridian.

The steam of mugwort has been used medicinally in many cultures. The herb was chopped into small pieces and boiling water poured over it. A pregnant woman or one with troublesome menstruation or uterine discomforts would sit or squat over the steam to ease her pain and relax her mind.

Finally, to round off the impressive benefits of mugwort smoke, it is a good insect repellent, including for clothes moths. Indeed this may be an ancient use, and some authors believe 'mug' in the common name is an old word for insect. In this sense 'wort' would be the herb that was effective against insects.

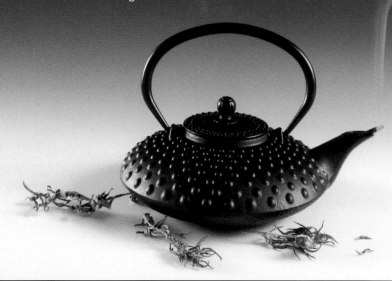

Mugwort **Rice**

Mugwort adds a lovely flavor to rice, with the dried leaves being more aromatic than fresh ones. In Japan each spring sticky rice is pounded with fresh Japanese mugwort, *yomogi* (*Artemisia princeps*) leaves to make vivid green mochi, which is then often stuffed with a sweet red bean paste. Similar recipes are popular in Korea.

We prefer to harvest our mugwort when it has silvery flower buds, before the tiny flowers open. Pick the top foot or so of each branch and dry in a dehydrator or on a drying rack in a dry place. When dry, the leaves and buds can readily be broken off the stalks, which can be kept to use as kebab sticks. The dried mugwort will keep in an airtight jar until you dry more next year, or have eaten it all.

Simply place **a small handful of dried mugwort** on top of your **rice** before steaming or boiling it. Follow the instructions for the type of rice you are using. Sticky rice (also called glutinous rice) works well, but you can use any type of rice you like. Wholegrain brown, red or black rice will take longer to cook than white rice.

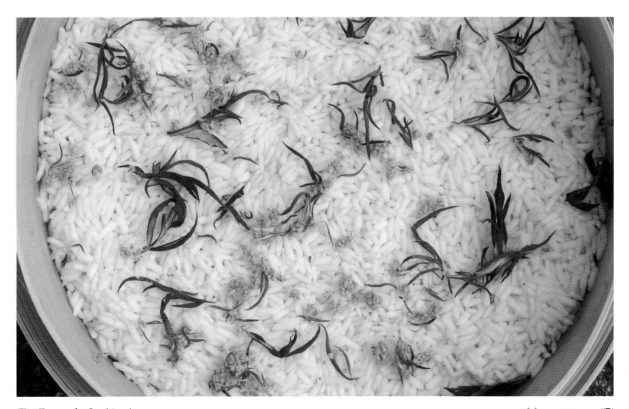

Mugwort-Smoked Kebabs

This recipe uses mugwort-smoked tofu and mugwort stalk kebab sticks for a wonderful flavor. Use your usual steamer but without any water.

To smoke the tofu, place **mugwort buds or leaf stalks** in the bottom of a steamer or pasta pot (photo below left). Cut **a packet of firm tofu** into cubes, and place them on the steamer above the mugwort (photo below right). It's helpful to use a glass lid, so that you can see how much smoke is being created. Heat gently.

The tofu will take on a mugwort flavor even if there is no smoke visible, but for a stronger flavor increase the heat a little to get some smoke. Taste the tofu after about 15 minutes to see if it is smoked enough for your taste, if not, continue smoking until it is.

To assemble the kebabs, strip the leaves off **6 or 8 stalks of mugwort**. Skewer the tofu, alternating with your choice of other vegetables. Here we used **yellow summer squash**, **cherry tomatoes**, **cubes of aubergine (eggplant)** and **button mushrooms**.

Brush with **olive oil**, or use your favorite marinade. Bake at 175C/350F for 15 minutes, or grill until done.

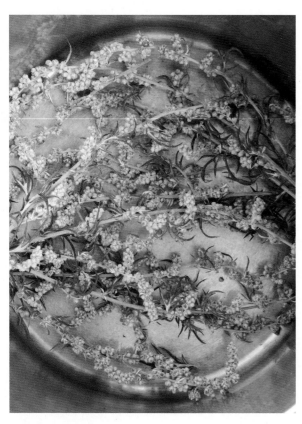
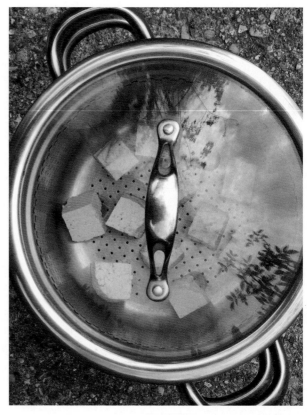

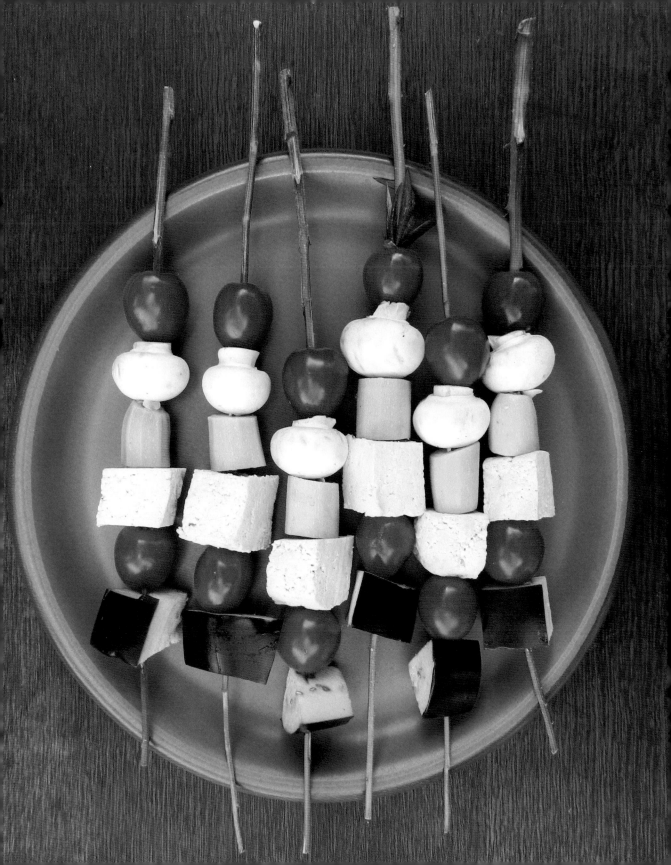

Mugwort & Mushroom **Soup**

Mugwort seems to enhance the flavor of mushrooms and works well in a soup.

Sauté   **150g (1 cup) chopped onion and shallot**
         300g (10 oz) fresh mushrooms, chopped

Add **500ml (2 cups) water**
Cook for 15 to 20 minutes.

Add
225ml (1 cup) oat or coconut cream
¼ teaspoon nutmeg or mace powder
a handful dried mugwort, crumbled

Simmer for a few more minutes. **Salt** to taste.

Makes 4 small bowls or two big ones.

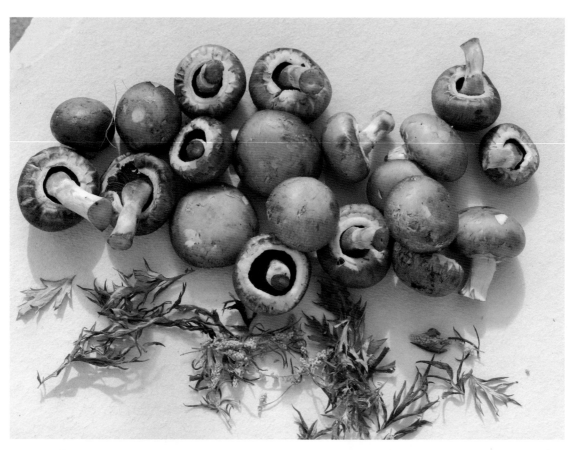

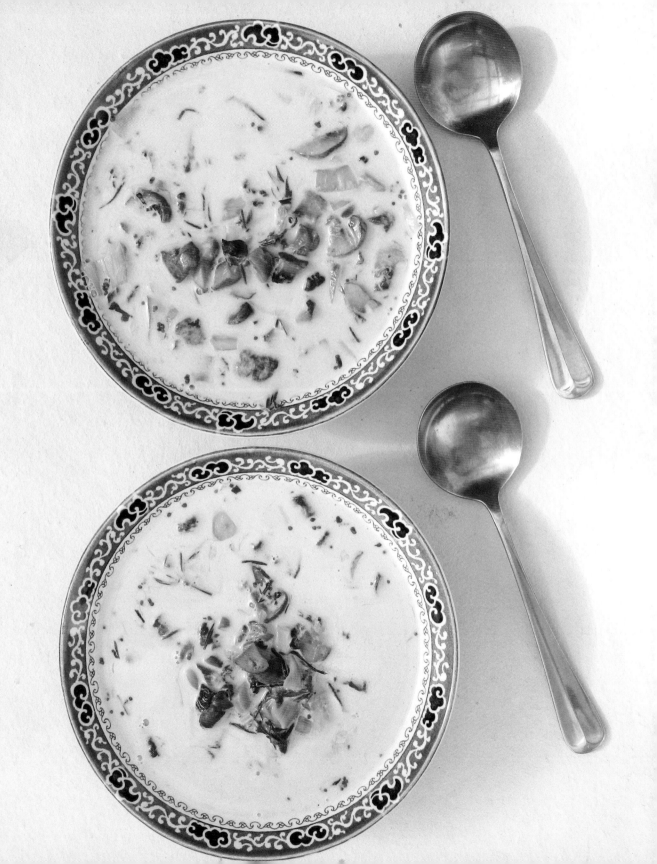

Mugwort & Lemon **Kefir**

Water kefir is easy to make, and is a healthier alternative to soft drinks, being full of beneficial micro-organisms and natural ingredients. The symbiotic colony of bacteria and yeast (SCOBY) that make kefir, form transparent pea-sized pieces, called grains.

Fermentation is in two stages, using the SCOBY for the first stage, then straining the grains out and adding flavorings for the second fermentation, which develops the carbonation or fizz.

You don't need to sterilize anything, but just make sure the containers you use are clean.

For the first distillation, put these ingredients in a large jar:
2 liters (4 pints) filtered or spring water
100g (½ cup) golden unrefined or demerara sugar
4 tablespoons water kefir grains or SCOBY

Leave for about 2 days. Warm weather will speed up the fermentation, and cold weather will slow it down.

Strain out the grains and save them for your next batch of water kefir. If you aren't ready to make another batch, store them in a jar in the fridge (with a couple of teaspoons of sugar and enough water to cover them) until you want to use them. Pour the liquid into a large jug or stainless bucket.

In a large saucepan put:
10g dried mugwort
1 liter (2 pints) of water
2 lemons, finely sliced or chopped up
50g (¼ cup) light brown sugar

Put a lid on the pan. Bring to a boil and simmer for 15 to 20 minutes. Remove from heat and leave to cool with the lid on.

When cool, strain the liquid and add it to the kefir, then pour into bottles. Latch-top bottles are best, but you can use bottles with a screw cap. Just remember to release excess pressure after a day or two especially in warm weather, as the build-up of pressure can eventually explode bottles if they are left unattended.

Leave for two days or until the liquid is as bubbly as you would like. It is then ready to drink, but can be stored in the fridge for a few days before drinking.

Alternatives: Water kefir can be flavored with almost anything for the second fermentation. You can add elderflower cordial or a few blackberries. We often use apple juice and then add other flavors, like some dried ground ivy or lavender. You don't need much to give a good flavor. Experiment and have fun!

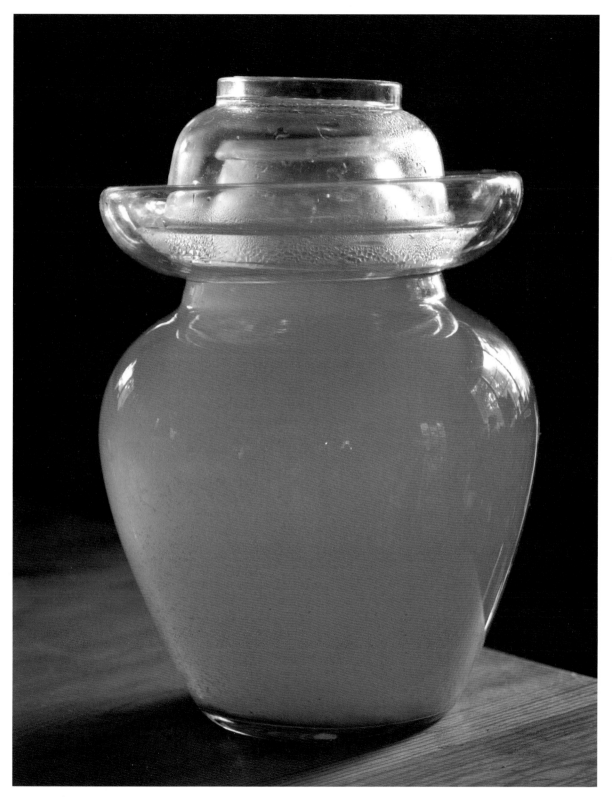

Nettle

Nettle (*Urtica dioica*) is one of our 'desert island' plants, offering us a pharmacopoeia of herbal medicines, compost, cordage and increasingly our food. If blackberry is our king of weeds in this book, nettle must be the emperor for its amazing variety of uses, including many recipes. If you don't have your own nettle patch in the garden, we advise you to make one or allow one in.

Urticaceae
Nettle family

Perennial.

Edible parts: young leaves and tops are best in spring, but will grow fresh when cut back.

Distinguishing features: Very familiar colony-making and perennial weed of farmland, woodland, gardens or river banks wherever there is a high-nitrogen soil; dark green hairy and stinging jagged leaves ascending in serried rows; insignificant tiny flowers and hanging bunches of seeds later; tough and aggressive yellow roots.

Edible relatives: *Urtica urens*, small nettle, a common annual, is similar in appearance and used in homeopathy; *U. pilulifera*, Roman nettle, probably introduced to Britain by the colonizing Romans, as a spinach-like food or reputedly to beat the flesh, is now rarely found.
The deadnettles are unrelated mints (*Lamiums*).

What kind of a weed is nettle?

All-conquering might be the response here. Nettle (*Urtica dioica*) prospers in nitrogenous soils in temperate and subtropical regions. While growing to about a meter, three feet or so, tall in Eurasia and North America, species in Nepal can be double that height, while Australia and New Zealand have a nettle tree (*Urtica ferox*) with huge spines – a science fiction nightmare.

'Stinging' differentiates nettle from its cousins, the deadnettles (*Lamiums* in the mint family), 'dead' referring to their harmless hairs. In Britain we have white, pinky-red and yellow wild deadnettle species, also charmingly known as archangels. Their flowers are edible and sometimes sucked by children for their sweet nectar. We have never really found the leaves good eating, but some foragers like them.

Everybody wonders why nettle needs its stings to defend it. The 20th-century naturopath Dr Vogel (1989) explained that nettle is so valuable that browsing animals would long ago have eaten it to extinction: *Animals, with their instinctive knowledge of what is good for them, would not leave us even one leaf.* Given this, it is good to know the sting is quickly disarmed by gentle heat, including cooking.

Nettles are wind-pollinated, which means they need no showy, fragrant flowers to attract insects. *Dioica* in the species name stood for 'two houses', giving 'dioecious' to describe its separate male and female plants. In reality, most nettle plants have male, female and hermaphrodite flowers. Seeing the pollen explode out of the male flowers is a wonderful, if unusual summer experience.

Its roots are another formidable weapon in nettle's spread and dominance. The tangled yellow roots with their long and strong fibers are tough, fast-growing and go deep. You should use gloves if you want to pull them out in the garden to avoid being comprehensively stung.

The roots readily put up new shoots and later decay as the new clonal plant becomes independent. Nettles are thus perennial, if not almost immortal. The effect is a dense colony, which further crowds out competitor plants from germinating.

The accessible minerals pulled up from the soil by nettle's deep roots are a good reason nettle is acclaimed for herbal use and for eating. We have all heard about the minerals and vitamins in nettle but it is also a surprisingly good source of wild protein (20% or more by weight) and fibers.

A factor in nettle's spread is its liking for (and by its own decomposition further adding to) nitrogenous soils,

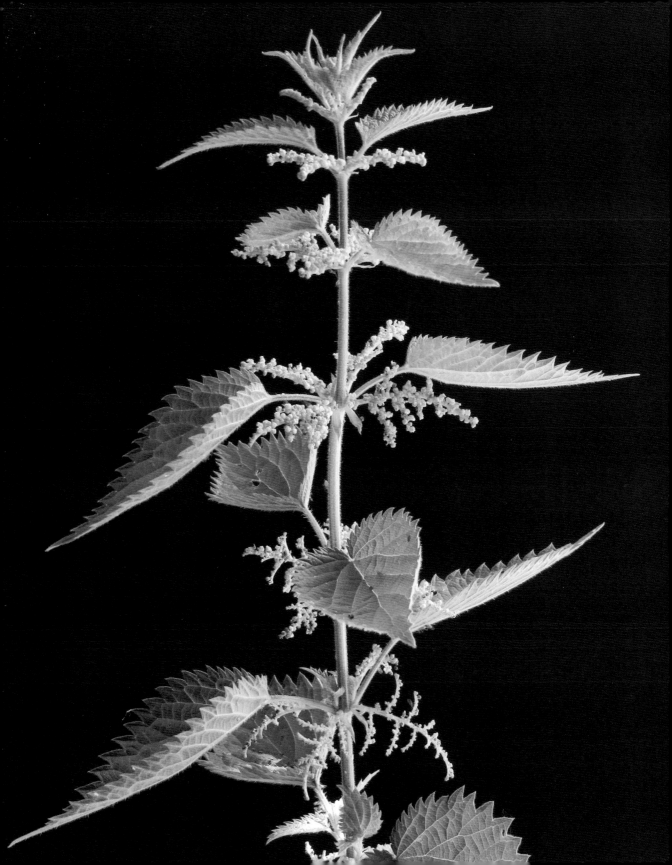

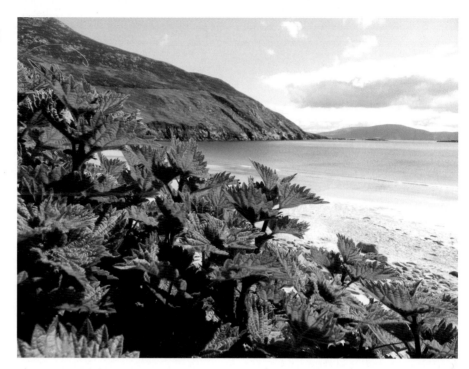

Nettle is also a weed of the shore: a view of Achill island, Co. Mayo

often associated with human waste. A nettle colony can thrive for hundreds of years, making it a marker for archaeologists: nettles in a landscape indicate past human activity, so dig here!

The history of nettle

Wind-pollinated plants like nettle leave problematic evidence in the geological record, but it is highly likely that their history preceded the last Ice Age.

Every western herbalist for whom we have surviving writings, from Hippocrates (c460–370BC) and Theophrastus (c371–287BC) onwards, mentions nettle as food and medicine.

It is known to be important in both ancient and modern Chinese, Egyptian and Ayurvedic (Indian) medicine.

The English name may be from Anglo-Saxon *noedl*, needle, either for the sting or nettle's use as thread. By AD725 it appears as *netlan*, by 1200 it was *netle* and by 1400 it was *nettle*, underlining its early presence in everyday life. The Latin family *Urtica* is from *urere*, 'to

burn'. As *wergulu*, nettle was a sacred herb of the Anglo-Saxons.

Nettle has been food and medicine for so long that its history is inseparable from that of culture as a whole. But there is a precise date when one of its best-kept secrets was unlocked.

The herbalist John Parkinson could only speculate in 1640 that 'the haire or rough downe' caused nettle's sting. By 1655, the scientist Robert Hooke had explained the exact mechanism in his book *Micrographia*.

Using a magnifying glass Hooke experimented on himself, stinging his arm and viewing the process. The sting was revealed as a rigid hollow tube or a 'Syringe-pipe'. It pierced the skin and 'served to convey' a 'corrosive penetrant liquor' across from the nettle.

He did not know the later chemical names formic acid, histamine and acetylcholine for the 'liquor', but Hooke had resolved the method. So, when we hold a nettle stem and run a hand from its base to tip, in one direction, this flattens the trigger syringes but doesn't activate them as happens when we crush them.

Julie impresses people on our workshops by nipping off the top leaves of a nettle, rolling them in a ball and chewing them, without harm. She knows her Hooke, that's all.

Herbal & other uses of nettle

Nettle is one of the world's major medicinal herbs, actively benefiting our respiratory, digestive, urinary and glandular systems.

In this space we can hardly do justice to a treatment range from anemia and arthritis to urinary problems and vitamin supplements. But, in brief, we can consider nettle as three medicines in one, the roots, tops and seed.

The **roots**, as a decoction (boiled tea) or tincture (with vodka), are known for treating prostate problems, and infections and inflammations generally.

The **tops**, as a tea, soup or dehydrated nettle juice powder, make an excellent spring tonic, and address anemia and gout, high or low blood pressure, coughs and allergies, skin problems, inflammations and high blood sugar, and regulate breast milk production.

The **seed**, dried, ground, then mixed into a paste with honey (the herbalist's electuary), can help stop bleeding, promote urine flow, treat burns and skin problems, be a kidney support, an energizer and an aphrodisiac.

As a product nettle has another vast range of uses. It is an ancient fiber plant, making cordage or ropes, woven into a fine, soft linen or a rough military uniform (as in Austria in the First World War). It makes a dye (leaves green, roots yellow), paper, sails, fishing nets, hair rinse and shampoo, insect repellent, a rennet…

How to eat nettle

Nettles are nutritious. Gardeners use them to feed other plants, adding uprooted nettles to compost or steeping them in water for a strong liquid fertilizer. Nettle leaves bring fruit to ripening, and were used to pack plums.

If nettles came from the Amazon or the Himalaya, they would be hailed as a superfood, but they are so common we take them for granted.

Nettles feed the caterpillars of several colorful butterflies, like the red admiral, peacock and small tortoiseshell, and many moths. When dried in hay, nettles are loved by cattle and other stock in winter.

Nettles feed humans worldwide and young leaves can be eaten year-round, though tender spring leaves are best. As in tea-picking, two leaves and a bud is a motto for nettle gathering, with the bonus that in a few weeks there is a fresh harvest of new, succulent leaves.

Use rubber gloves to pick the leaves (the sting is strong in spring) or simply use scissors to cut and lift them into your bag or basket. Gathering extra allows you to freeze them for future

Sage soup, east or west
Two sages are renowned for eating quantities of nettle soup and literally turning green for their pains, but also enjoying long lives: St Columba in Scotland (AD521–597) and Milarepa in Tibet (AD1052–1135). The first dish is still eaten as St Columba's broth and the second as *satuk*, nettle soup.

Colcannon cream
Cyril and Kit Ó Céirín (1978) quote an old Irish song that extols colcannon (creamed greens, including nettle): *Did ye ever ate colcannon that's / Made from thickened cream, / With greens and scallions [onions] blended / like a picture in your dream?*

We saw these cows at Malham Cove, Yorkshire, eagerly munching the local nettles. They had probably read their Dr Vogel (p178)!

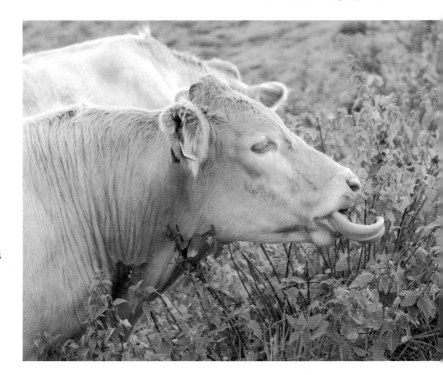

use: blanch in boiling water for two minutes, drain and cool, then store in freezer bags.

It is worth stressing that it's best to gather your leaves before the nettles flower. Young spring tops are best, and by cutting your nettles back you help encourage fresh growth later. Nettles in the shade will be milder and juicier than those in hot sunny places.

Nettle leaves either fresh or dried and crumbled are universally boiled as a soup or borscht.

Ray Mears and Gordon Hillman (2007) tested a **nettle seed** soup, but found it too burning in the mouth or stomach. We suggest sticking to the leaves.

Nettle kail remains a Scottish nettle soup, eaten for Shrove Tuesday or spring in general, with nettle added to barley or oatmeal, plus onion or wild garlic. In west Yorkshire, spring or Lenten dock pudding features oatmeal, bistort and nettle leaves, again with onion or wild garlic.

Nettle porridge can be made like the soup but with extra oatmeal. Samuel Pepys's diary from February 1661 records his enjoyment of this meal. Nettle is also an ingredient in haggis.

The old name poor man's spinach conjures up other recipes. Adding cream in some form always enriches the overall taste of 'greens'.

There are infinite nettle recipe possibilities, with two recent takes we have seen being nettle leaf curd and nettle sauerkraut. We give recipes for various savories, and a cake and banana bread; we could have added smoothies, tea or beer.

Any drawbacks? Some people object to a urea (fertilizer) smell when nettles are cooked or when the leaves take on a darkish color from the weight of chlorophyll (to keep leaves bright green, blanch before cooking). The flavor is fairly mild, so can easily be disguised by using spices if you wish.

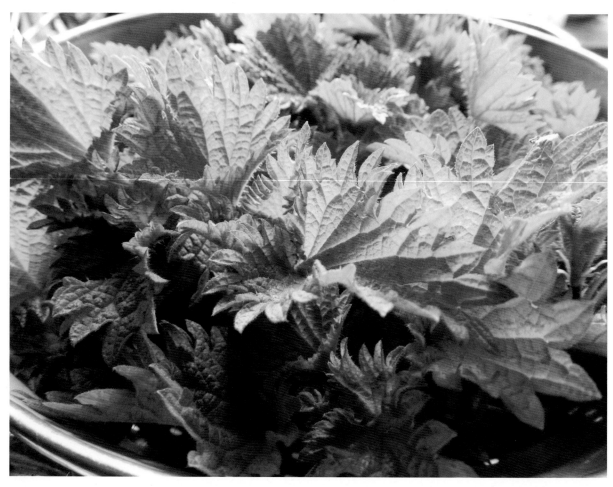

Nettle **Purée**

This nettle purée is a starting point for all sorts of nettle recipes, including the vibrant green cake on the next page. Blanching the nettles ensures they keep their lovely bright color.

Pick **a colander full of nettle tops** – this will be about 100g. Rinse them if they need it. Cook for a few minutes in a little **boiling water**, just until they look soft. Strain off the brownish cooking water to use in something else (add to soups and stews for extra nutrition). Rinse the nettles with cool water to stop the cooking, then gently squeeze out the excess water.

Put it in a blender with **125ml (½ cup water)**, then whizz it all up until smooth.

This purée can be frozen for later use. Freeze all together for the cake recipe or use an ice cube tray for small amounts that can then be added to soups, sauces or other dishes. A cube or two blended with a banana, the flesh of an orange and apple juice makes a tasty superfood smoothie that will kickstart your day.

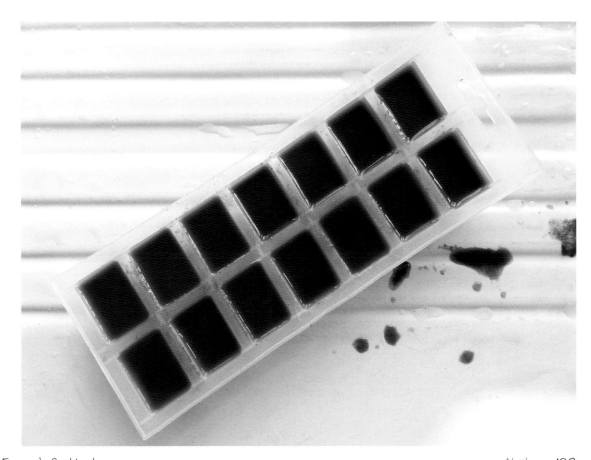

Nettle Cake

This cake is a gorgeous bright green color. Preheat the oven to 175C/350F.

Cake
Heat gently in a pan until soft:

1 tablespoon vinegar, 50g (2 tablespoons) golden syrup or maple syrup, 4 tablespoons olive oil, 4 tablespoons coconut butter, and **130g (1 cup) soft light brown sugar**

Beat well and stir in **1 cup nettle purée** (see p183)
Sift **240g (2 cups) unbleached white flour** and mix into the batter.

In a cup, pour **1 tablespoon boiling water** onto **1 teaspoon baking soda (bicarbonate of soda)**

Pour into batter and stir well. Pour batter into 2 greased and floured 20cm (8in) cake pans.

Bake at 175C/350F for about 25 to 30 minutes, until the cake looks done and an inserted straw comes out clean.

Cool on a rack before removing the cakes from the tins.

Trim off the top of one of the layers, if necessary, to make it flat.

Lemon icing (frosting)
Beat to a cream:

250g (2 cups) icing sugar (confectioner's sugar)
125g (½ cup) vegan butter or coconut butter, warmed to soften
juice of half a lemon
finely grated zest of half a lemon

Spread a layer of icing onto the bottom cake before placing the other cake on top. Ice the top and sides of the cake, using a spatula or a piping bag. In the facing picture I've used double the quantity of icing as a special treat.

Decorate with edible fresh or crystallized flowers, such as violets, violas, primroses or lilac.

Alternatives:
We sometimes double the recipe to make 4 layers, or three layers of cake and some cupcakes.

You can use any icing or topping that you like. If you want it less sweet, try draining thick coconut yogurt in a jelly bag; rest this on a sieve over a bowl for half an hour to remove excess water. Add vanilla extract or other flavoring to taste and spread on the cake. Keep the cake chilled.

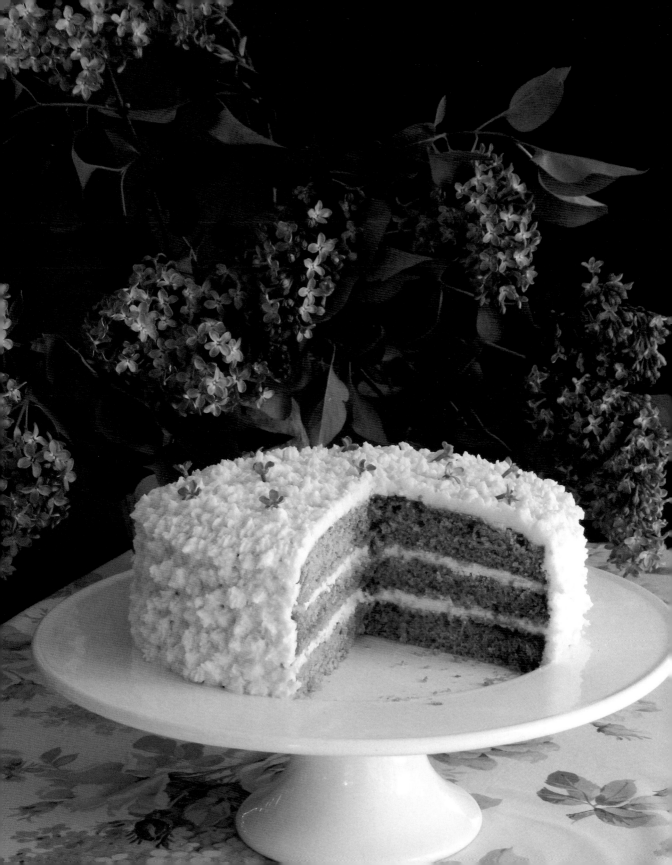

Nettle Crisps

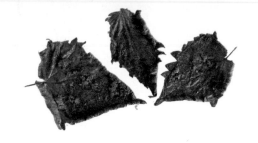

Nettle crisps have a crunchy, satisfying texture and are a really quick way to make a wholesome, healthy and moreish snack.

You need **medium-sized nettle leaves**. Gather a handful or so for your first experiment and vary the amounts as you prefer.

Check the leaves carefully for aphids and butterfly eggs (on the underside) and discard any if need be. Be aware of the sting, which will, rest assured, disappear in the cooking. You can, however, get stung while gathering, so take care.

Wash the leaves, ready for your dipping sauce. You will need about 4 tablespoons of sauce.

Blend **toasted sesame oil** (or any cooking oil), **some flakes of nutritional yeast**, **pepper** and **salt**. We had intended to use paprika but added **sumac** instead, a lucky improvisation.

The oil and the yeast are the heart of the taste and the condiments are refinements. The sauce should be of a paste consistency and is so umami that any green leaf tastes good in it.

Dip your leaves in the sauce, making sure both sides are coated, and put them on a baking tray. Bake in a medium oven for a few minutes until they are crisp. Keep your eyes on the progress of the crisping as it can quickly go too far and you end up with a burnt offering.

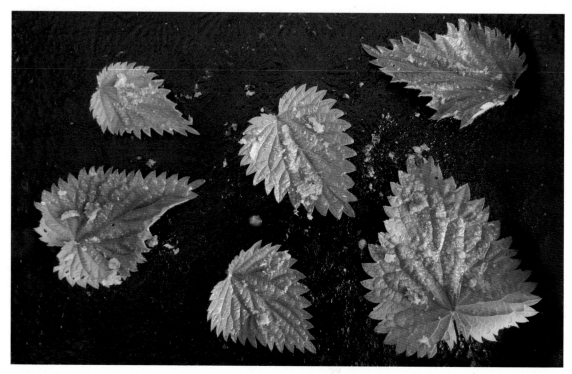

Nettle **Risotto**

Nettle makes a great risotto, because the chopped leaves hold up well to lots of stirring without disintegrating. We like to make our own stock, with potato peelings, carrot and celery scraps etc. You can use stock powder if you are short of time, but take care it's not too salty. This risotto takes about 30 minutes to cook. Serves 4 to 6.

Heat about **1¼ liters (5 cups) of good vegetable stock.**
Keep it warm while you make the risotto.

Put in another saucepan **4 tablespoons olive oil** and **1 largish onion, finely diced**. Cook until the onion becomes transparent, then add **2 teaspoons dried marjoram, 2 cloves minced garlic** and a **pinch or two of nutmeg powder**.

Stir well, then add **400g (2 cups) Arborio or other risotto rice**. Stir to coat in the onion and oil mixture, and cook for a few minutes, until the rice grains look translucent. Then add **125ml (½ cup) white wine** and simmer and stir until the wine has mostly been absorbed.

Add up to a cupful of the hot stock, stirring. When the broth has been mostly absorbed by the rice, put in another cupful, stirring each time you add liquid. After adding the fourth cup of broth, put in **1 cupful of chopped, blanched nettles (about 50g)** and start tasting the risotto. It needs to be cooked through, *al dente* or a little chewy, but not mushy. Add the last of the stock if needed. When it's cooked to your taste, remove from the heat and stir in **juice and finely grated zest of half a lemon, ½ cup yeast flakes** and **salt and pepper to taste**. Serve immediately, loosening with a little broth if needed, and drizzle with a little extra olive oil.

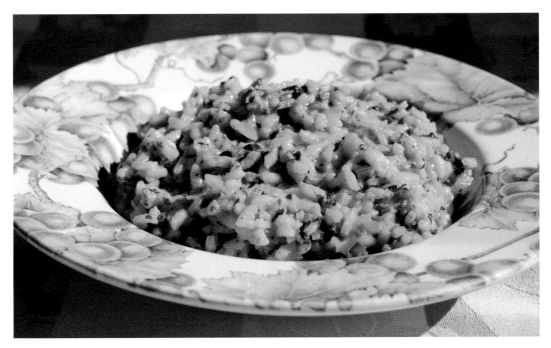

Nettle Tagliatelle

Fresh pasta always tastes so much better, and it is suprisingly quick and easy to make.

For 2 people: **80g (½ cup) semolina (farina)**
                        60g (½ cup) pasta flour
                        pinch of salt
Slowly add **4½ to 5 tablespoons nettle purée**.

Mix until the dough holds together in a ball. Knead until smooth. Let rest for half an hour.

Roll out. Use a pasta machine to roll to setting 5, then run through the Tagliatelle setting. Or roll thinly by hand using a rolling pin, and cut into 1cm-wide strips. Hang them on a rack to dry so they don't all stick together while you boil the water. If you don't have anything to hang them on, just lay them on the kitchen table with a dusting of flour to stop them sticking.

Cook the strips in **rapidly boiling salted water** for 3 minutes (or a minute or two longer for thicker noodles – taste to see they are done). Serve with your favorite creamy sauce or with oil and garlic.

Alternatives: The pasta dough can be shaped any way you like, to make ravioli, tortelli, tortellini or lasagne, etc. If you don't have pasta flour, use all semolina.

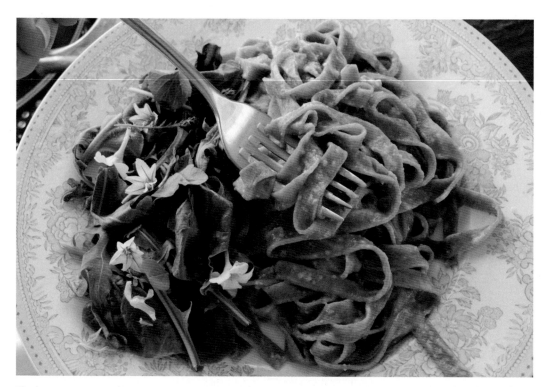

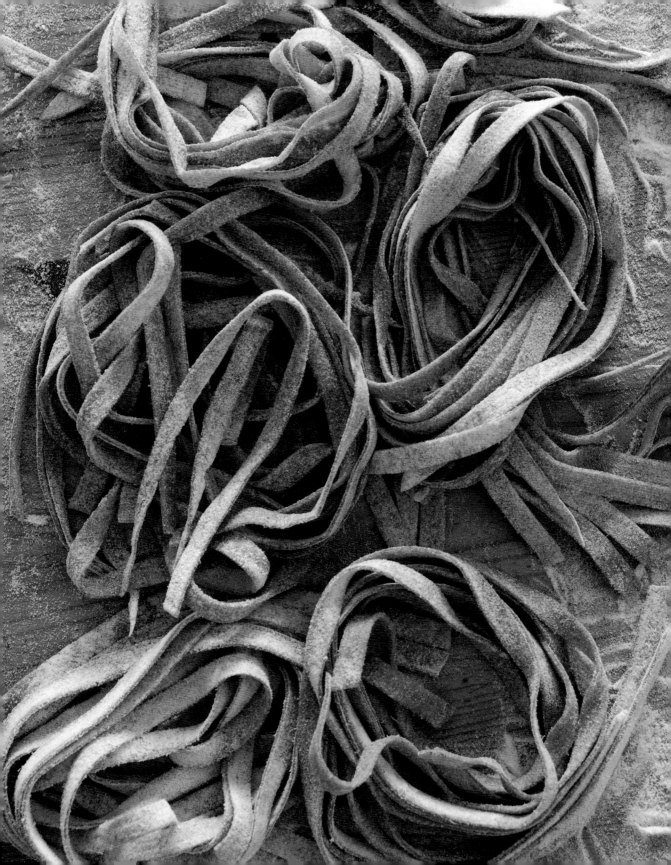

Nettle Bannock

This is a type of soda bread similar to those popular in Ireland. Julie's mother often used to make soda bread when camping, because it was not only delicious, but quick and easy to do and it could be cooked in a lidded frying pan, without any need for an oven – though we do use one for this recipe. It has a delicate pale green color, with a real added nutritional boost from the nettles.

Mix together:
450g (4 cups) wholemeal (wholewheat) flour or malted bread flour
180g (1½ cups) plain (all-purpose) flour
1½ teaspoon bicarbonate of soda (baking soda)
1 teaspoon salt
200ml nettle purée (see p183)
200ml soy milk
2 teaspoons cider vinegar

Knead the mixed ingredients on a lightly floured surface until smooth. Place in an oiled skillet. Use a knife to mark into 8 pieces. Bake at 200C/400F for about 45 minutes, or until golden on top – it should sound hollow when tapped.

Serve warm. Can be eaten at breakfast or any time of day. Goes well with soup, such as the one on the facing page.

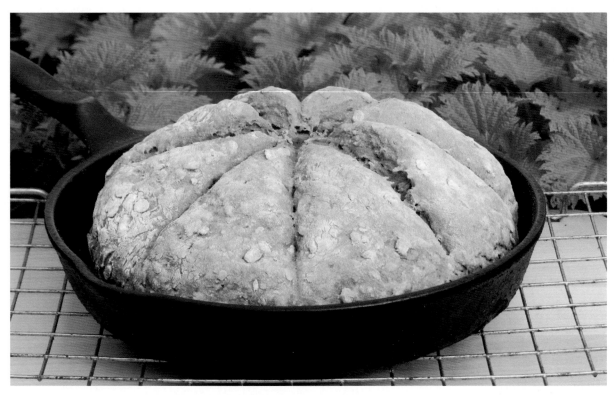

Nettle & Pea **Soup**

Many people already have their own favorite spring nettle soup recipe, but we find this very simple recipe using peas is particularly tasty.

Blanch **a colander full of nettle tops**. Rinse in cold water and drain.

Put the nettles in a blender with 250g (**2 cups) of thawed frozen peas** and **950ml (4 cups) vegetable stock** (or use **water** and add **2 teaspoons boullion powder**) then pour into a saucepan and heat gently.

Alternatives: If you want your soup a bit thicker, add **35g (¼ cup) gram flour** (or chickpea/garbanzo flour) mixed with **120ml (½ cup) water**. Heat, stirring until it thickens and the gram flour is cooked.

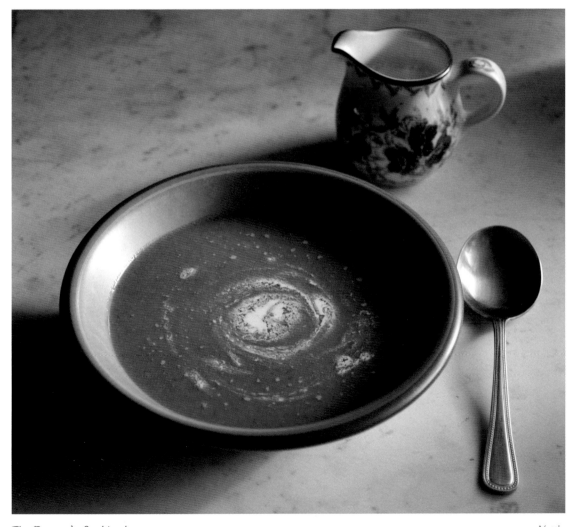

Nettle Saag Aloo

Saag is an Indian term for greens, usually taken to be spinach or mustard greens, but here we have used nettle leaves. Saag aloo is greens cooked with potato and spices.

Simmer about **1kg (2¼ lb) potatoes**, cut into chunks, until just tender.

Heat **2 tablespoonfuls of vegetable oil** in a large saucepan. Add **2 teaspoons cumin seed** and **2 teaspoons mustard seed** for a minute or until they start to sizzle.

Add **1 onion**, chopped. Cook until soft and beginning to brown. Add **3 garlic cloves**, crushed and a **3cm (1in) piece of fresh ginger**, finely chopped or grated. Cook for 5 to 10 minutes, then add the cooked potatoes and stir to mix.

Add **250g (½ lb) nettle leaves**, blanched and chopped. Cook for another 5 or 10 minutes.

Serve with rice and poppadums, and daisy raita (p68), ground elder bhajis (p119), sowthistle bud pakora (p231) or any other Indian dishes you like.

Alternatives: Nettles can be partly or wholly replaced with many of the other greens in this book. Fat hen, orache and sowthistle work particularly well.

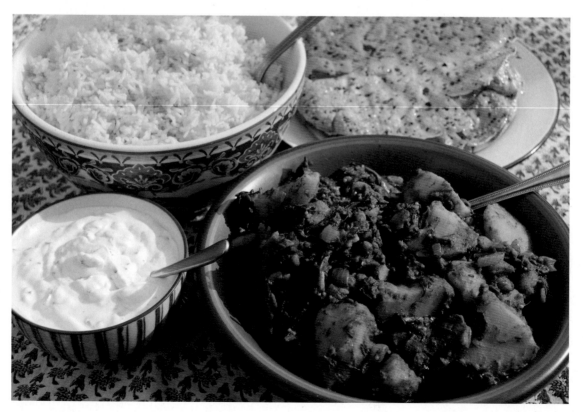

Nettle Banana Bread

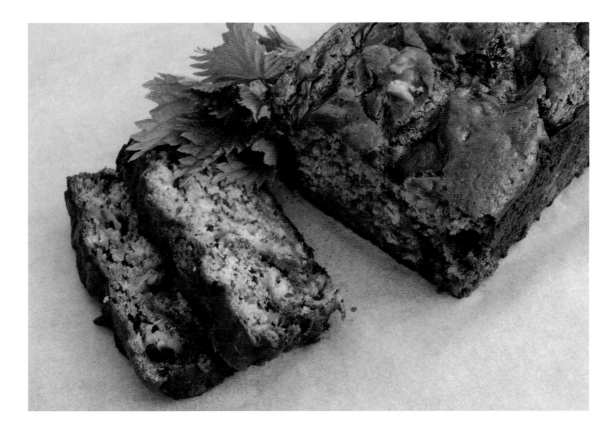

This marbled banana bread is moist and delicious, with ribbons of bright green running attractively through it. It is quick and easy to make as below, or with gluten-free flour. Preheat oven to 175C/350F.

Mash **4 very ripe bananas** (about 1½ cups when mashed). Mix with **100g (½ cup) demerara sugar, 2 tablespoons sunflower seed oil or other vegetable oil** and **80ml (⅓ cup) almond milk or water**.

Add **180g (1½ cups) flour, ½ teaspoon bicarbonate of soda (baking soda), ½ teaspoon baking powder** and **½ teaspoon salt** to the banana mixture. Stir to mix.

Scoop out **125ml (½ cup)** of this mixture, and mix with **125ml (½ cup) nettle purée** (see p183).

Grease a loaf tin. Scoop in alternate half cupfuls of the two mixtures. Take a butter knife to swirl patterns through the batter. Don't overmix or it will all look the same!

Bake at 175C/350F for 55 minutes. Let cool before turning out of the tin.

Nipplewort

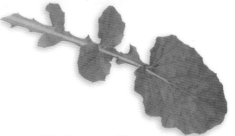

Nipplewort (*Lapsana communis*) has a life beyond its highly specific common name, and is a 'wort', a healing plant, which has also earned a forager's reputation as a tasty wild green. To offer some variation on the usual boiling and serving with oil, our recipes have borrowed from various cuisines in the form of a nipplewort gremolata, tabbouleh, a spring soup and oriental dumplings.

**Asteraceae
Daisy family
(formerly Compositae)**

Annual.

Edible parts: Leaves before flowering almost any time of year; buds.

Distinguishing features: A rosette of leaves through the winter and early spring. The leaves are soft, hairy and blunt-ended, with one large and many smallish lobes. The flower spike is tall, to 1m (3.3ft) or more, slender, open with multiple branches; flower buds are nipple-like; flowers small and pale yellow, sow thistle-like; no pappus (parachutes) on seeds; non-latex sap (i.e. sap is clear, not white like dandelion sap).

What kind of a weed is nipplewort?

Nipplewort (*Lapsana communis*) announced itself to us a few summers ago when it seemed to be taking over our garden. Like most people, we hadn't thought about it much, but we did wonder if it was telling us something.

A member of the vast Asteraceae family (think daisy or dandelion), nipplewort is plain and functional rather than beautiful, though the pale yellow flowers are lovely in close-up and the leaves pleasingly green.

It is a ruderal species, these being settlers on waste land (the Latin original term means 'rubble'), but also likes disturbed soil – hence it is a weed of both arable fields and our gardens.

An unusual fact about it is that the flowers only open in the mornings of sunny days. Forager Miles Irving (2009) goes as far as saying, *flower heads that open much after 10am on sunny days are probably not nipplewort.*

It is hardy, though, and grows quietly through the winter, with its flat rosettes of basal leaves appearing early in the year. These develop firm roots in order to push up the lanky stems, which can reach over a meter (3.3ft) high.

The flowerhead is sow thistle-like, but unlike dandelion, it has no pappus (parachutes) or milky sap, though it does have a small amount of clear sap.

Lacking the means of flying away, young nipplewort seeds settle mostly close to their parents, earning their common name *communis* or social. It grows quickly and produces numerous seeds, viable for about five years.

Of course, the main thing people want to know about this plant is its unusual name. Here there is a mystery. Is nipplewort so named because the flower bud looks somewhat like a small nipple, and then people used it to treat nipple pain?

Was it an example of the 16th- and 17th-century **doctrine of signatures**, in which God was thought to have made a plant look similar to the problem it could treat, like a lungwort to treat the lungs? Or was this plant so specific to treat nipple pain that it took that name?

In our opinion, the bud isn't particularly nipple-like, and a dandelion, to take one close relative, might be better suited to the name. On the other hand, nipplewort retains a folk reputation, however earned, for treating swollen breasts.

The history of nipplewort

There are occasional records of nipplewort in archaeological sites around central and northern Europe

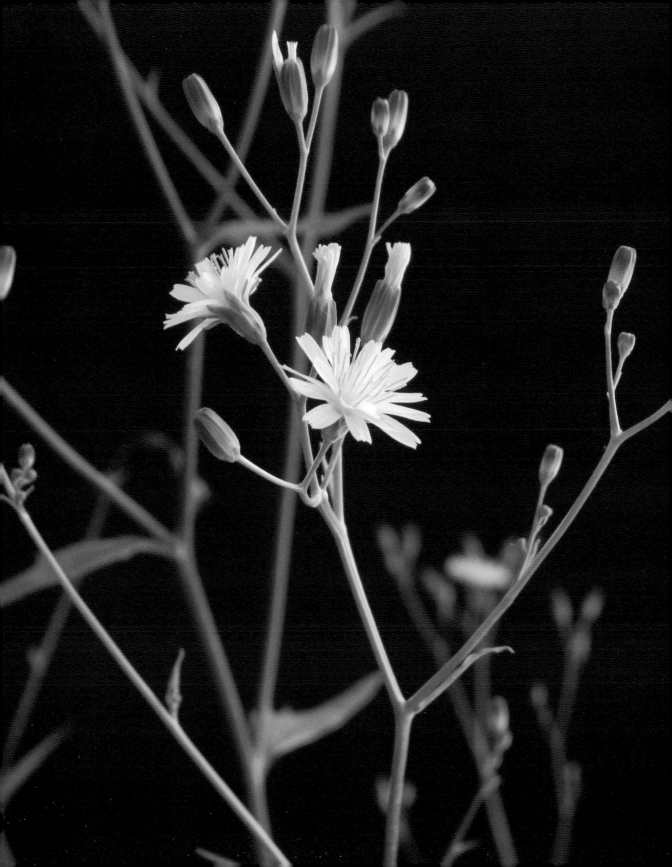

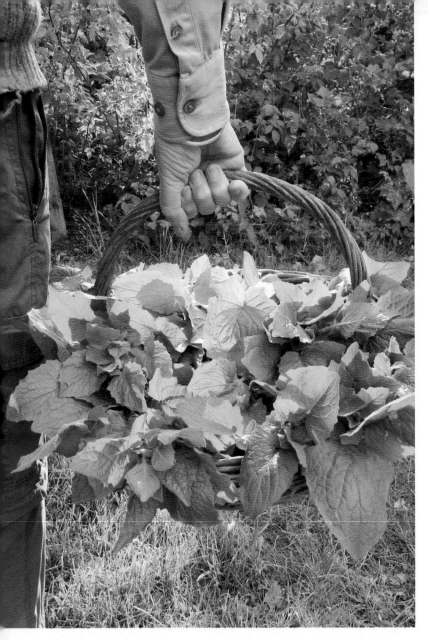

The green man (actually Matthew in his green shirt) with his basketful of basal-leaf nipplewort for lunch

Fifield Bavant, Wiltshire, UK, and in Vallhagar, Sweden, while the last meal in the stomach of Grauballe Man, in Denmark, from the same period included nipplewort as well as many other seeds.

Presence of seeds, however, is not a firm indicator of a plant's use: they could be the remnants of a meal, as in the Grauballe man, or incidentally occurring weeds of the time. But the physical seeds nonetheless seem to offer firmer evidence than the writings from the Roman period that followed.

The best-known Roman story concerning nipplewort refers to the civil war between Pompey and Caesar. The siege of Dyrrachium (modern Durres in Albania) took place in 48 BC, and Caesar's troops complained they were getting no wages and had to eat the roots of 'lapsana' But was this nipplewort?

Lapsana (or lampsana) is indeed the modern scientific name for nipplewort, a daisy family species, but history and hazy botany obscure the exact identity of the Dyrrachium plant.

Some commentators propose white charlock (*Sinapis arvensis*) or wild radish (*Raphanus raphinastrum)*, both cabbage species, while the first-century AD naturalist Pliny called *lapsana* a 'hairy white cabbage'. He added that when cooked it 'soothes and relaxes the bowels'.

In none of these cases, however, would the roots be substantial enough to be collected and eaten by an army as famine food. And if it was the leaves that were used, as you might expect, why didn't the sources say this?

Perhaps the best thing to emerge from this confusing tale is the comment about 50 years after the battle by the writer Plutarch, who reports the troops making loaves from the *lapsana* – whatever it was – by mixing milk with the flour and the leaves. It's an idea for a modern nipplewort bread, perhaps.

in the Neolithic period, starting about 8,000 years ago.

Nipplewort was one of many wild Compositae plants that accompanied the development of agriculture, as woods were cleared and wild species, like barley, wheat, rice, mustards and cabbages, were bred as food crops.

Closer in date, there are Iron Age findings from roughly 2,300–2,500 years ago, for example, in sites at

There is no particular wealth of medieval reference to nipplewort as either food or medicine, but Joachim Camerarius the Younger (1534–98), a German botanist and physician, wrote of it in 1586 in his *Hortus medicus et philosophicus* (The medical and philosophical garden).

He reported that apothecaries in Prussia prescribed the herb, known there as *Papillaria*, to soothe and heal women's breasts. John Parkinson, our favorite English herbalist, picked up on this in his *Theatrum Botanicum* (1640) by giving the plant its first English name, nipplewort.

Modern herbal writers David Allen and Gabrielle Hatfield (2004) shrewdly note that such a late coining of a common name *suggests in turn the use* [of the plant] *may have been a late infiltration into the folk-repertory of Britain.*

Certainly it was known to folk medicine in Scotland, its name, according to Geoffrey Grigson (1955), being Bolgan-leaves, with bolgan meaning a swelling. The larger basal nipplewort leaves are recorded as used as a breast poultice by nursing mothers.

Herbal & other uses of nipplewort

Parkinson admitted that he knew of no herbal uses – *We have no properties to shew you of this Lampsana* – but offered an opinion that nipplewort might be *temperate in heate and drinesse, with some tenuitie* [sharpness] *of parts able to digest the virulency of those sharpe humors that break out into those parts* [nipples].

We can infer that the treatment might be administered as a poultice, ointment or tea. These are the ways we use it, though occasions have been few.

The modern herbal commentator who has followed up most is Julian Barker (2001). He suggests nipplewort is laxative but soothing to the gut, while its ointment can offer some relief in the chronic condition of pruritis ani, or scratching of the skin around the anus.

He also says nipplewort is diuretic and can be helpful in cases of oliguria or renal insufficiency. Further, the leaves are hypoglycemic and might be used in treatment of mature-onset diabetes.

Julie found for herself that drinking nipplewort tea countered a bout of lightheadedness induced by too much bending over and adopting awkward positions while photographing plants in a Cairngorms meadow. Perhaps nipplewort has an unresearched role in improving low blood pressure?

How to eat nipplewort

Nipplewort is an open, branching and sparse plant whose basal leaves are relatively substantial but whose upper leaves taper towards the top. The basal leaves, before it sends up a flower stalk, are mild and taste like lettuce. Thereafter, the leaves become bitter.

They are easy to gather, but tend to hold dirt on the slightly hairy surface, so make sure to wash them well.

Camerarius [1586] *saith that in Prussia they call it* Papillaria, *because it is good to heale the Vlcers of the Nipples of womens breasts, and thereupon I have entituled it Nipplewort in English.*

– Parkinson (1640)

The young and tender leaves of this vegetable have the flavor of radishes, and may be eaten raw, as salad. Though possessing a bitter taste, they are a wholesome vegetable; and, in some parts of England, the country people boil them as a substitute for greens.

– Domestic Encyclopaedia (1802)

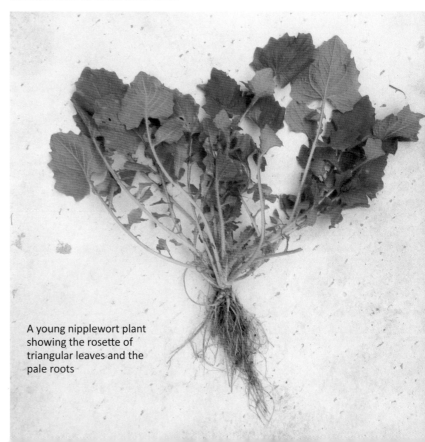

A young nipplewort plant showing the rosette of triangular leaves and the pale roots

A template for pretty much all wild greens, including nipplewort, is to find means to temper their tendency to roughness or bitterness. The key message is to pick the young leaves, in spring, before the plants need to become more fibrous so as to support the flowers and seedheads.

If eating raw, try adding lemon juice plus a strong herb taste such as parsley and garlic in some form. If cooking,

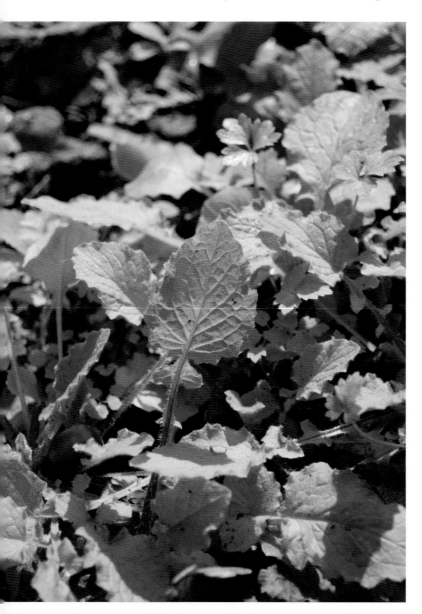

some foragers like to boil the greens for 10 minutes, then discard the water and reboil with fresh, before frying or baking the blanched leaves.

The plain young leaves of nipplewort are tasty and mild by themselves in winter and spring, or cooked in hearty stews, soups and casseroles. They wilt quickly, so it's best to use them immediately after picking.

Our gremolata recipe opposite is a nipplewort-based take on the Italian *salsa verde* and could be the base for South American *chimichurri* sauce.

A specifically Japanese nipplewort species, *Lapsana apogonoides*, forms part of a millennium-old tradition to welcome in the new year.

Seven young types of greens are customarily gathered for a spring herb soup, eaten on 7 January. The time-honored ingredients are Japanese parsley, shepherd's purse, cudweed, chickweed, turnip and radish in addition to the nipplewort.

We like spring soups, and have adapted the Japanese recipe to what is weedy and on hand in our English garden. We chose seven ingredients, and in the soup pictured (p205) we feature nipplewort as the main green presence, with a mix of wild garlic, nettle, chickweed, Jack by the hedge, dandelion and ground elder.

We also prepared millet, as a tribute to the Japanese recipe, to add gluten-free virtue and substance, along with miso and soy sauce. Buckwheat noodles would be an alternative choice for people on gluten-free diets.

A Zanzibari cornmeal dish and a Lebanese-style tabbouleh, then a Japanese dumpling recipe to serve to display the international cuisine credentials of nipplewort.

And, as an extra idea, there's always the historical nipplewort bread that the Romans just might have made at the siege of Dyrrachium.

Nipplewort **Gremolata**

Gremolata is a traditional Italian *salsa verde* (green sauce), with varying ingredients but usually containing parsley, garlic and lemon. We have substituted nipplewort leaves for parsley, and it remains delicious as a flavorsome sauce to go with any savory dish, or try a dollop in your soup. It can be made with other green spring weed leaves, and use orange in place of lemon if you want a sweeter, less piquant experience.

Chimichurri is a similar South American green (or red) sauce, which substitutes wine or other vinegar for the lemon and adds red peppers and chilli.

30g (1 cup) fresh nipplewort leaves (use entire if still young, or chop if stringier)
2 garlic cloves
zest and juice of a small lemon
olive oil (roughly the same amount of liquid as the lemon)
salt and pepper to taste

Put all ingredients in your food processor and blitz for about 20 seconds. It's ready to serve and lasts a couple of days in the fridge (but probably less because you will have eaten it).

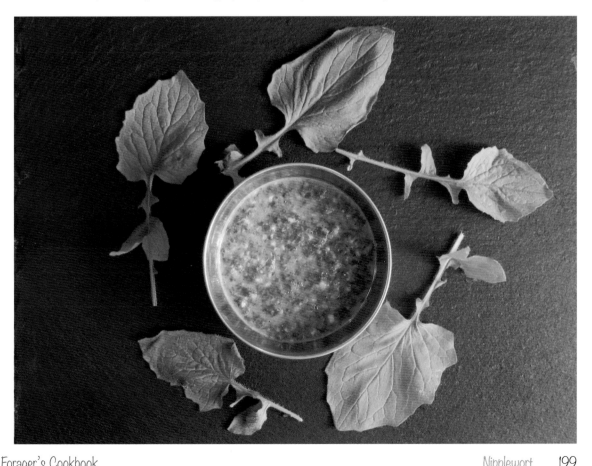

Zanzibari-Style Nipplewort

This recipe is delicious whatever greens you use, and is inspired by the delicate spicing of Zanzibari cooking. The flavors all meld to create something more delicious than the sum of its parts, and it's the perfect complement to polenta (yellow cornmeal). We'd go so far as to say this is one of our favorite recipes for cooked greens.

Chop **an onion** and fry gently in **a little coconut oil**.
When the onion is becoming translucent, add **½ teaspoon nigella seed (black seed or black cumin)**, **½ teaspoon turmeric powder**, **½ teaspoon cardamom powder** and **1 or 2 cloves garlic, crushed**.

Fry gently for a few minutes
Add **200ml (¾ cup) coconut milk**
about **200g nipplewort or mixed greens** (a colander full)
and **a cup of chopped tomato** (we like to use cherry tomatoes, halved or quartered, for their flavor)
Add **salt and pepper to taste**.

Cook gently for 10 or 15 minutes.

For the polenta, boil **1 liter (1.76 pint) of water**, and add **1½ teaspoons salt** and **200g polenta (yellow cornmeal)**, whisking to remove lumps. Put a lid on and cook gently until done (or follow instructions on your cornmeal – precooked types take hardly any time).

When the cornmeal is done, spoon it into a large serving dish or 4 individual bowls and make a hole in the center. Spoon the greens mixture into the hole and serve.

Alternatives: If you don't have cornmeal, this recipe can also be served with cooked rice, millet or other grains. Nipplewort can be combined with or replaced by fat hen, orache leaves, spinach, or most edible greens.

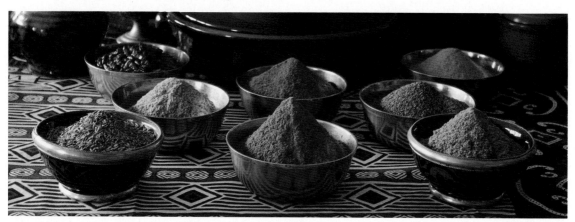

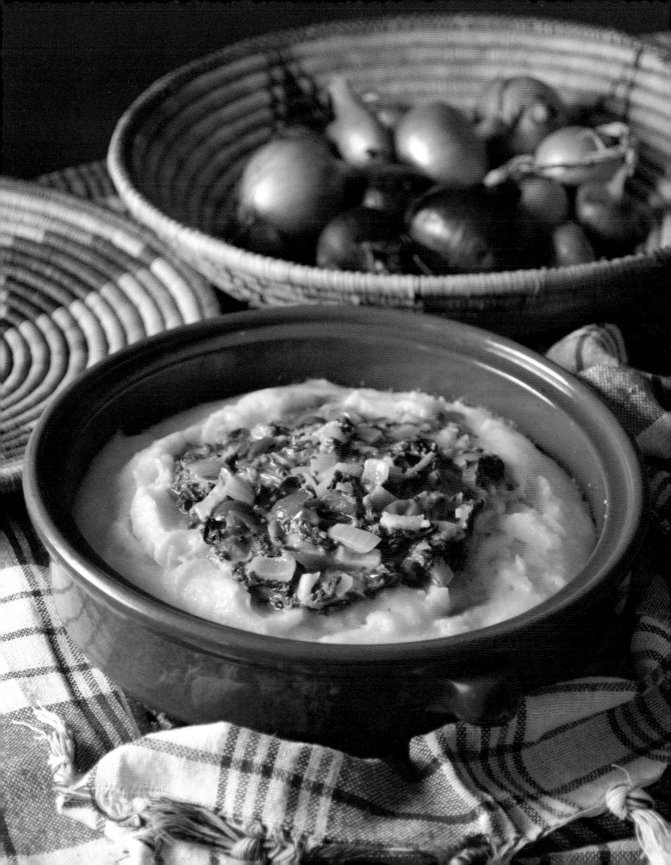

Nipplewort **Tabbouleh**

Nipplewort replaces the parsley in this Lebanese-style tabbouleh salad. It's a hearty salad that can be a meal on its own, or served alongside a main meal or as part of a selection of hot and cold mezze. Serves four.

Mix together **120ml (½ cup) boiling water** and **50g (¼ cup) bulghur**. Add **1½ onions, finely diced**. The heat of the water removes the sharpness of the onions. Let stand for 20 minutes.

Then add **1 teaspoon salt**, **¾ teaspoon cinnamon**, **½ cup fresh lemon juice**, **¼ cup olive oil**. Chop **500g (1¼ lb) tomatoes**, **2 handfuls fresh nipplewort** and **a small handful fresh mint** to the mixture.

Taste and add **salt, pepper** and **lemon juice** and some **lemon zest** to taste. Leave in a cool place for an hour before serving, so that the flavors can meld.

Alternatives: Decorate with edible flowers if you like – we use ground ivy flowers, chives and wild garlic in the spring. You can also combine the nipplewort with other greens.
Use spring onions (scallions) in place of chopped onion, but add them once the bulghur has cooled so they keep their bright green color.

To make a gluten-free version, replace the bulghur with cooked quinoa.

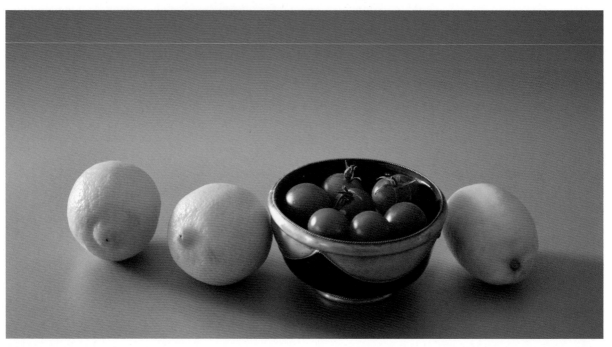

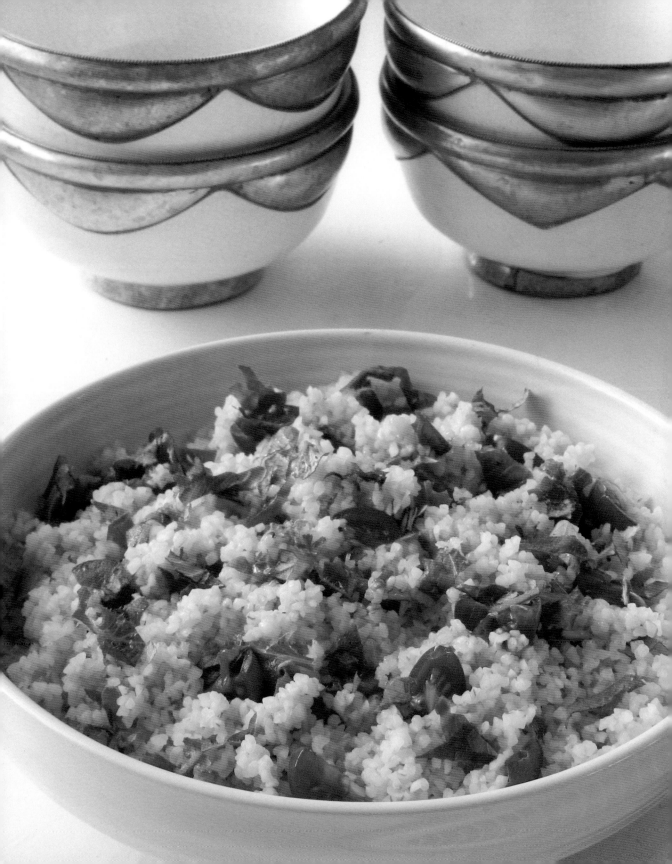

Nipplewort Spring Soup

This soup is inspired by the seven herbs revered in Japan as part of the celebration of spring, using equivalent tastes in herbs more local to us, with nipplewort at the center of the recipe.

Pick **2 good handfuls nipplewort leaves**. Remove the tougher stems and chop.

Pick **1 good handful of other spring leaves (we used wild garlic, nettle, chickweed, Jack by the hedge, dandelion and ground elder)**. Remove the tougher stems and chop. Set the greens aside.

In a large saucepan, fry **1 clove of minced garlic** and **1 finely diced shallot** in **a little oil** until transparent. Add **100g (3½oz) diced firm tofu** and cook a little longer to brown the shallot.

Add **1 liter (1¾ pint) vegetable stock** or water and **1 tablespoon ginger**, freshly grated.

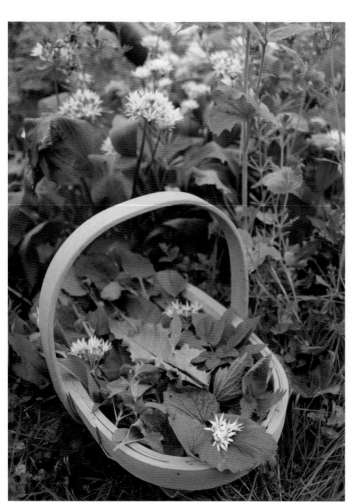

Heat until simmering, then add the prepared greens and cook for about 5 minutes.

Add **1 tablespoon miso** dissolved in **a little water** and **soy sauce to taste**.

Pour into two soup bowls.

Garnish with **black sesame seed** and **wild garlic or chive flowers**, and with **a drizzle of toasted sesame oil**.

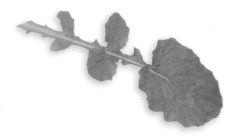

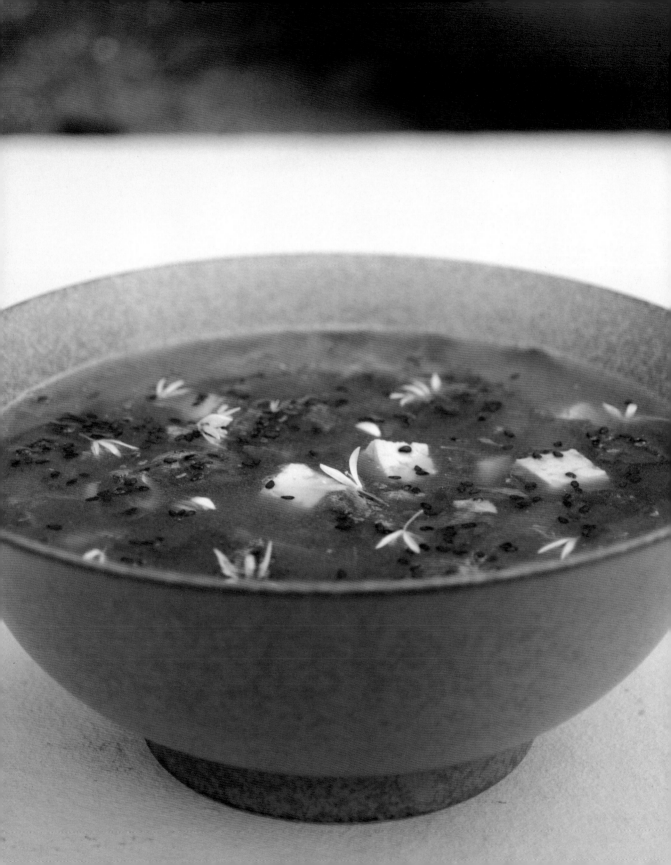

Nipplewort Gyozu/Jiaozi

These oriental dumplings are quite elegant, but are simple to make. The filling can contain almost anything, but we enjoy the taste of nipplewort. Chinese dumpling flour gives the best results but if you can't get it, use ordinary flour. Makes about 20 dumplings.

Put **180g (1½ cups) dumpling flour** in a bowl, and make a well in the center. Pour in **125ml (½ cup) hot water** (almost boiling). Mix well – it should be fairly dry. Knead into a smooth dough that doesn't stick. Add **a little more hot water** if you still have dry bits after kneading for a minute. Rest the dough in a covered bowl for half an hour while you make the filling.

Fry **150g (1 cup) finely diced shallot or onion** and **2 or 3 cloves minced garlic** in **a little toasted sesame oil** until translucent. Add **60–90g (2 or 3 cups) chopped nipplewort leaves or mixed greens** and **2 teaspoons grated ginger**, cooking until the nipplewort has wilted. Mix in **250g (1 cup) mashed smoked tofu** (use bought smoked tofu or smoke your own – see p172).

Take a ball of dough about the size of a walnut – you should have enough for at least 20. Flatten with your hand, then roll outwards from the center with a rolling pin, turning as you go. Your finished circle should be 1 to 2mm thick (slightly thicker towards the middle), and about 7 or 8cm (3in) in diameter. Use **a little flour** if they are sticking. We had a dumpling press to shape ours, but you don't need one. Put a spoonful of filling in the middle of each circle of dough, then wet the edges by dipping your finger in **water**. Pleat the edges together with your fingers or by pressing in the dumpling press. Steam for 15 minutes or until cooked.

Dipping sauce: Mix in a small saucepan **165ml (¾ cup) water, 2½ tablespoons tamari, 1 tablespoon white balsamic vinegar (or rice wine vinegar), 1 tablespoon maple syrup** and **1 tablespoon cornstarch.** Heat gently and stir until the sauce becomes clear and thickens.

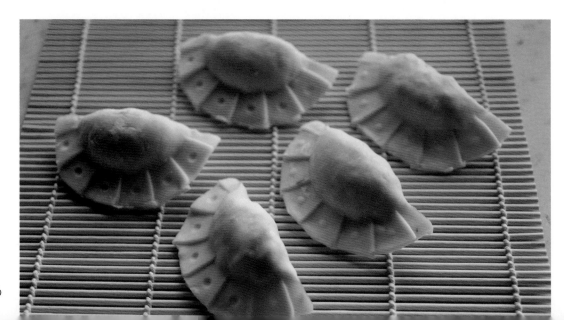

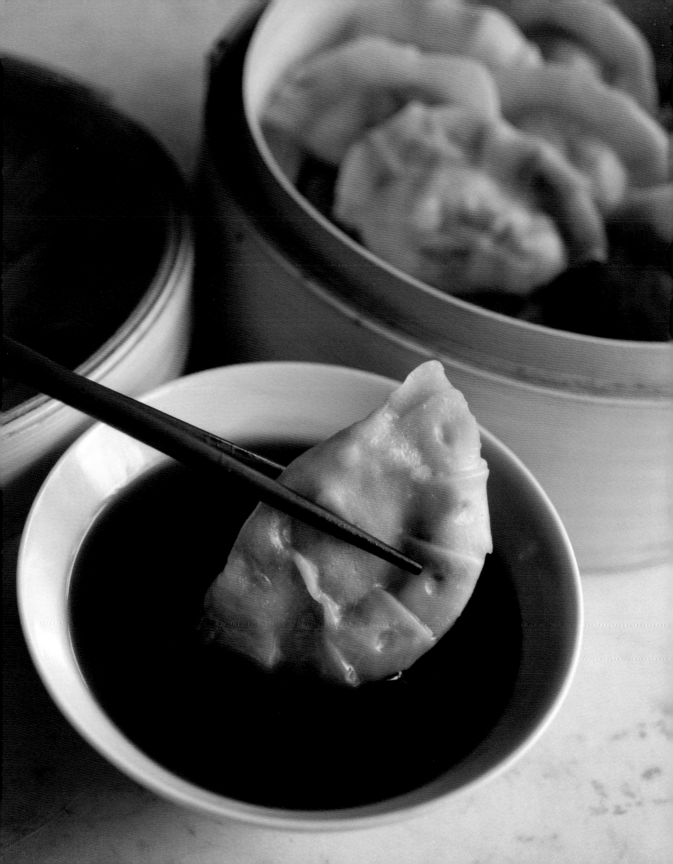

Plantain

Greater or broad-leaf plantain (*Plantago major*) and ribwort plantain (*P. lanceolata*) are common weeds of footpaths and lawns, and have followed European settlers around the temperate world. Best known as first-aid remedies for stings, bites and cuts, they also offer under-appreciated foraging opportunities.

**Plantaginaceae
Plantain family**

Perennial. Greater plantain can sometimes be annual.

Edible parts: Buds in late spring to autumn, young leaves, seeds in autumn.

Distinguishing features: The habitat chosen by **greater or broad-leaf plantain**, of compacted or trodden soil, is challenging and, by growing *in* the path, it has few weed competitors. Its wavy-edged, rather messy broad leaves with long stalks and tight, slender 'rat's-tail' flower spike are characteristic.

Ribwort plantain likes areas *just next to* the path. Its long, narrow, deeply veined leaves, black flower buds and circle of white stamens on top of a tall stalk are defining features.

Edible relative: Buck's horn plantain (*P. coronopus*) is grown as a vegetable in Italy where it is known as minutina or erba stella.

Right: ribwort plantain, the backlighting revealing the lengthwise leaf veins, long flower stalks and fuzzy flowerheads, as well as the plant's communal habit

What kind of a weed is plantain?

The genus *Plantago*, with about 270 species worldwide, is named from *planta*, Latin for sole of the foot. Greater plantain is shaped like a rounded foot and, like ribwort plantain, will flourish where human or animal feet have compacted the earth.

Plantains' niche on or by footpaths reduces competition from other plants. As fast-growing perennials, they reach almost a meter (3 ft) tall in the case of ribwort, when undisturbed and in richer soil, and half that in *P. major*.

The leaves have firm ribs, with fibrous strengthening tissues that make eating unappetizing when the plant is old. Indeed, the fibers were once used for weaving and string-making.

Part of the success of the *Plantago* genus is high seed productivity. Salisbury (1961) estimates that *P. major* can yield 15,000 seeds per plant, with high germination rates (60-plus percent) and good durability (dormancy of up to 40 years).

The seeds pass unharmed through the digestive system of a bird, animal (and human) eating them and can launch a new colony. Plantain seed cases are slightly mucilaginous when wet, sticky enough to attach to a passing deer or rabbit, and be spread that way.

Note: the banana family of edible plantains (*Musaceae)* is not related.

The history of plantain

Plantago species, usually as seeds, feature widely in European archaeological sites. Two 'bog' bodies from Iron Age Sweden and Denmark, so-called Tollund and Grauballe man, dating to some 2,400 years ago, had plantain seeds in the stomach.

At much the same time in China, the first herbal compilation to survive there, *The Yellow Emperor's Classic of Internal Medicine*, referred to *Che qian zhi* (*Plantago asiatica*) – in English translation 'before-the-cart seeds'. It remains part of the modern Chinese pharmacopoeia.

About the same time in Greece another emperor, Alexander the Great, used plantain root to cure headaches.

Pliny the Elder's *Natural History*, from the first century AD, claimed that plantain has 'marvellous virtues' as an astringent, a wound herb and for rheumatism.

Putting a leaf or two of any species of *Plantago* in the shoe or sock was long believed to ease hot and tired feet and to treat plantar fasciitis, a painful inflammation of the fascia (or connective tissue) on the sole between the heel and toes.

Plantain was *waybroed* (waybread) to the Anglo-Saxons. Its status was very high, as 'mother of plants' and one of the nine sacred herbs; in these pages

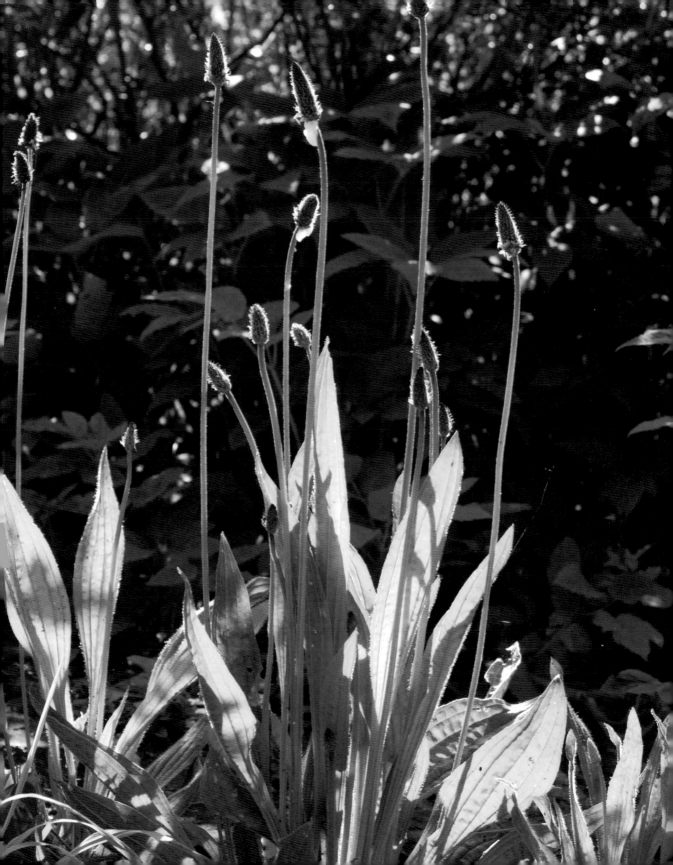

And you, Weybroed,/ mother of plants/ open to the east, mighty inside:/ Over you creak wagons,/ over you rode women,/ over you rode brides,/ over you snorted bulls./ You withstood all/ and offered resistance./ So withstand the venom/ and contagion/ and misfortune/ that sweep across the land.
– Lacnunga, a 10th-century Anglo-Saxon leechbook

The presence in this plant of tannins, mucilage, silicic acid and glycosides ensures a wound and pain remedy of the highest order.
– Holmes (1989, rev. 2020)

Maria Merian's engraving of greater plantain and its associated moth in caterpillar, pupal and flying stages, c1670

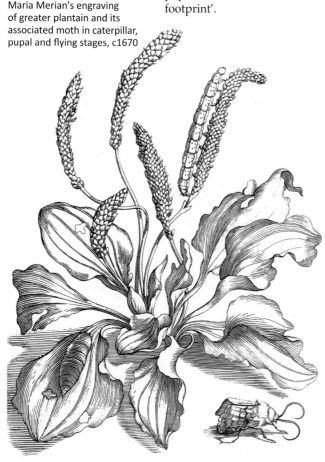

we also look at mugwort, nettle and shepherd's purse – all now 'weeds' rather than sacred.

All through the ancient civilizations of the temperate world – whether ancient Egypt, parts of India or Latin America – plantain was present.

In Mexico, in the early 16th century, the Spanish found the Aztecs ate a gruel of *P. psyllium* (psyllium). Today, across South America, *el llanten* is a popular commercially sold plantain tea.

It was soon noticed that where the white man invaded or colonized, *Plantago* would follow. In North America and New Zealand alike, it had the popular name 'white man's footprint'.

In 1855 the American poet Longfellow publicized the idea in his poem-cycle 'Hiawatha' in these lines:

Wheresoe'er they [white men] *tread, beneath them / Springs a flower unknown among us / Springs the white man's foot in blossom.*

The foremost ethnobotanical survey of northwestern Native American peoples, by Nancy Turner (2014), describes a 'near universality' of plantain use and naming by local peoples in her study area, in over 20 languages and leading dialects.

This frequency suggests either that a species was already native or a very early introduction. Plantain was prized as an Indigenous burns treatment.

The likely native species in eastern North America is blackseed plantain (*P. rugelii*), named for a 19th-century German botanist, Father Rugel. It resembles *P. major*, with red–purple coloring on the leaf rosette, not green.

Herbal & other uses of plantain

Being plants of paths and roads as well as gardens and farms, plantains are readily available and recognizable around the world.

This ubiquity matters if you are in a strange place and need first aid for a nettle sting, a mosquito bite, a wasp sting, a boil or a burn – in fact any skin inflammation with painful heat, including eczema and varicose veins.

Such experience is cross-cultural: one Cherokee elder ironically called plantain 'Indian bandaid' (Garrett & Garrett 1996).

Treatment can be as immediate as a 'spit poultice': pick a plantain leaf, chew it for a few seconds and spread the bolus on the wound. The antihistamines and tannins present quickly reduce heat, neutralize poisons, stop bleeding and calm the mind.

A wad of plantain leaf in the mouth is good for toothache, while an old European protection against snakebite was to save a leaf in pocket or purse; a former American name for plantain was snakeweed.

The plant's energetic action is purifying, drying and drawing. Perhaps the best description was left by the 2nd-century AD physician Galen. His insight was that [plantain] *dries without biting or sharpness and clears heat without causing heaviness or stupefaction.*

Internally, the mucilage in the leaf, and especially the seeds, is soothing for the lungs, digestive tract and hemorrhoids. Hayfever and hot, dry cough, bronchitis, stomach ulcers, irritable bowel and constipation can also benefit.

As the seeds absorb moisture and swell in the stomach, they dry the tissues and soothe them. This is most true for *P. psyllium* (or *P. ovata*); in India this is a well-known Ayurvedic remedy for easing constipation and stopping diarrhea.

Taken with water, psyllium seeds quickly become a glutinous mash. Be cautious: because powdered psyllium absorbs so much liquid you need to keep well hydrated when using it.

Plantain can also absorb pollutants, with research ongoing about its potential in bioremediation of land made toxic by oil or heavy metal waste. This is a good reason to be careful where you harvest it for eating.

Modern medical research is actively investigating plantain's ancient reputation in cancer and diabetes treatments.

The leaf fibers, especially of greater plantain, have long been used to make string or used in weaving, and, like the bluebell, plantain was found to be sufficiently starchy to stiffen clothes when this was high fashion.

How to eat plantain

Plantain leaves make the best eating when young and fresh, before the fibers become stringy. Spring gathering encourages a second flush later on as the plant replenishes for winter.

The leaves of buckshorn plantain (*P. coronopus*) are a delicacy in Italy, and often grown in gardens. This plantain features in the Italian wild green salad *misticanza* or French equivalent, *mesclun*.

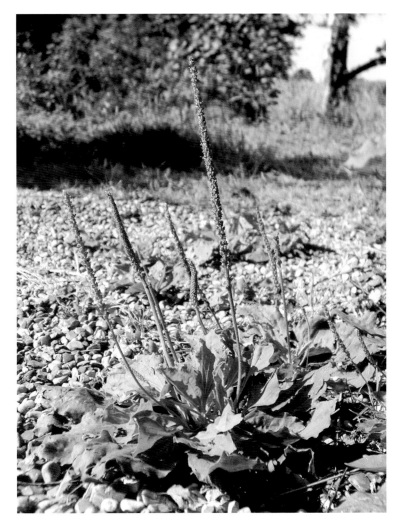

Greater plantain seeds are a handy wayside snack in autumn and early winter. Particularly in damp weather, the seeds and husks strip easily from the stems, and have a pleasant nutty edge.

Gather plantain seeds when ripe if you want to store them, picking entire stalks. Spread these on brown paper to dry fully before shucking off the seed cases that contain the individual tiny seeds; store these in brown paper bags or jars.

In Mediterranean cuisines, cooked plantain leaves were often served with yogurt and garlic, or stuffed with

Above: greater plantain, early summer, the crinkly broad leaves and 'rat's-tail' flower spikes flourishing in our gravel drive

I consider plantain to be one of my staple foods when I am on long hikes or walkabouts where I am only eating the wild foods around me. They make a perfect traveling snack and sustain me with energy; the seeds are packed with nutrients. – Blair (2014)

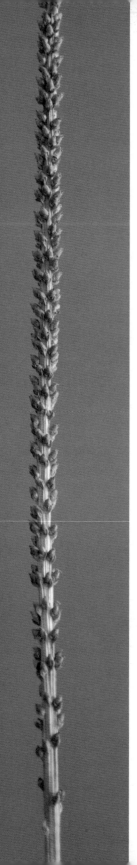

boiled rice, as is more often done nowadays for vine leaves. We like a simple garlic sauce spread on ribwort leaves (p215).

Broad-leaf plantain leaves reputedly have a mushroom flavor when boiled or sautéed, though this has eluded us so far. We sometimes add a leaf or two when we cook rice to give it a subtle but pleasant flavor.

It's easy to get excited, thinking of 'waybread', when you encounter elven bread (*lembas*) in *Lord of the Rings*. But, sadly, Tolkein's travel food didn't include plantain.

But has there been a tradition of bread made of plantain seeds? Very likely it has been done in the distant past, but it's a slow job to gather enough seeds, remove the husks and grind into a flour. Instead we have chosen to use ancient-grain flour to fashion waybread buns with a topping of greater plantain seeds and husks (p214). And we had no qualms in using a breadmaker.

An American forager/writer who eats plantain seeds literally as a waybread is Katrina Blair, whose book on wild weeds (2014) has an excellent chapter on plantain.

She writes of going on hikes on the Colorado Trail at 10,000 ft, relying only on wild food that she gathers on the way. She relishes raw plantain seeds, whether young and fresh or brown and nutty, finding the green, unripe seeds taste like 'a delicious green vegetable'.

The brown seeds do have a gelatinous mouth-feel but, as we have seen, this has its own benefits. Indeed, perhaps we should begin to think of plantain as a local and free form of chia seeds, with the same absorbent qualities.

Other cooking options for your fresh plantain leaves could include making crisps (as we do for nettle, p186), crackers (opposite page), a pesto (as we do for chickweed, p42) or a soup (as we do for nipplewort, p204).

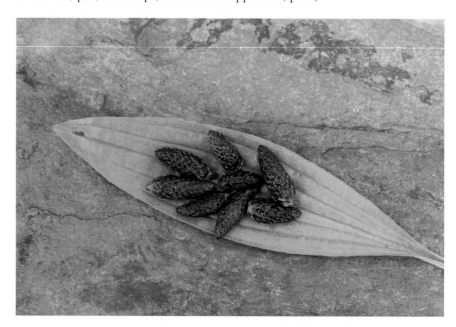

Left: greater plantain ripe seed stalk; above: ribwort immature flower buds

Waybread **Seed Crackers**

Plantain seeds and their husks are easily stripped off the stalks when they are ripe, as in the background image. Use fresh or dry and save them for later.

Preheat the oven to 160C/325F.

Mix in a bowl:
200g (1½ cups) sunflower seeds
100g (¾ cup) sesame seeds
75g (½ cup) flax seeds
35g (¼ cup) plantain seeds and husks
2 tablespoons psyllium husk
1 teaspoon salt
2 cups water

Leave to sit for about 15 minutes or until thick and gloopy. Line two baking sheets with non-stick greaseproof paper or silicone mats, and spread the mixture out thinly. Bake for an hour or two, rotating the trays if necessary, until the crackers are crisp. Leave to cool.

Break into pieces and store in an airtight container. The are delicious served on their own as a snack, or try them topped with a spread or served with a dip.

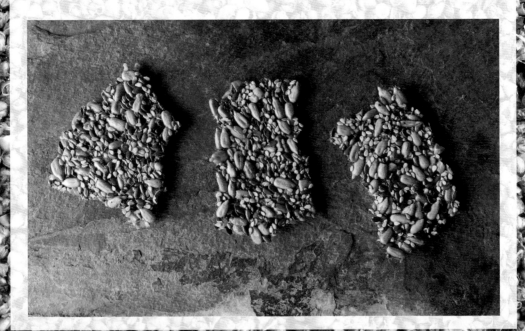

Waybread **Buns**

Put in a breadmaker or a large bowl **330ml (1⅓ cups) tepid water**, **½ tablespoon vegetable oil**, **1½ teaspoons of salt** and **1½ teaspoons of sugar**.

Add **570g (4¾ cups) of flour** (the illustrated buns used ancient grains, mostly emmer and einkorn with some spelt flour) and **1½ teaspoons of dried yeast** on top of the flour.

Turn the breadmaker to the dough setting and set it going, or mix by hand. When the dough is mixed, shape the buns into balls. Press the tops down into slightly flattened discs. Now sprinkle **dried plantain seed husks** on the buns, moistening the tops slightly if needed to keep them there.

Cover the buns with a teatowel, place in a warm place for 15–20 minutes to prove, then bake them in the oven for 10 minutes or until golden brown. We like them still warm from the oven.

Makes about 12 buns. The seeds taste nutty: an easy way to get your fiber!

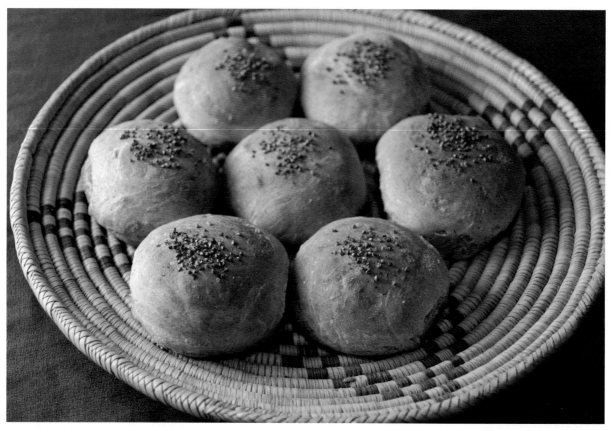

Plantain with **Garlic**

Set some **water** to boil and add **a little salt**. Wash **a handful of young ribwort leaves**, and place whole in the boiling water. The cooking time is important: you want the leaves to be boiled enough to be tender but not too much so as to be mushy. We find this to be about 4 minutes, but pick out a sample leaf any time after 3 minutes and see if it is tender; it may take slightly longer.

When ready, remove the leaves and place in **a bowl of cold water** for a couple of minutes. This will stop the cooking process.

Meanwhile prepare the sauce. Mix **1 tablespoon toasted sesame oil**, **1 teaspoon soy sauce**, **1 minced garlic clove** and **a teaspoon of toasted sesame seeds**. Add **salt** to taste.

Remove the plantain leaves from their cold bath. Toss together with the sauce in another vessel. Rest it all for a couple of minutes and serve as a side dish with rice.

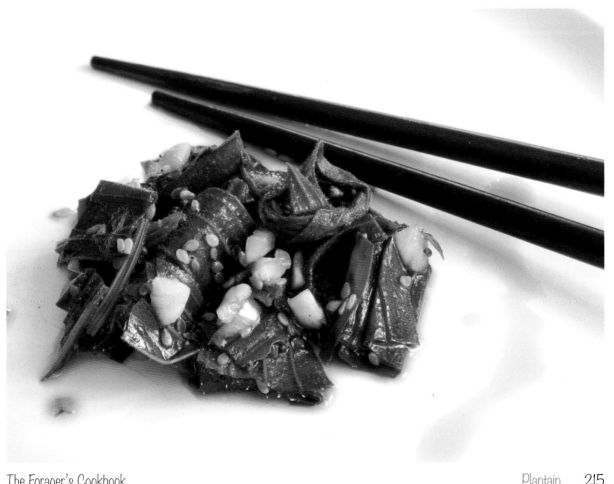

Sorrel

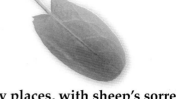

Sorrel (*Rumex acetosa*) is a common weed of lawns and grassy places, with sheep's sorrel (*R. acetosella*) being found in heaths and places with acid soils. Sorrel is a foodie favorite at present and often foraged for fine-dining restaurants. It comes with a long culinary history for its easily gathered sourness and was the 'lemon of the north', made into a greensauce, soups, porridges and possets before French sorrel and lemon itself usurped its role.

Polygonaceae
Knotweed family

Edible parts: Whole plant above ground, but mainly leaves.

Distinguishing features: Common sorrel and sheep's sorrel are perennial native plants across Eurasia, and introduced to North America and other temperate regions. **Common sorrel:** narrow and erect, to about half a meter (20in); stems hollow; arrow-shaped leaves, basal rosette with bottom lobes pointing backwards; topmost leaves smaller, clasping the stem; flowers tiny, orange-red, in clusters, followed by red fruits.
Sheep's sorrel: prefers wetter areas with acid soils, less common in gardens; smaller overall, with more open foliage; stems solid; basal lobes of leaves point sideways or forwards; upper leaves not clasping stem; flowers similar, even more rufus in color.

Edible relatives: French sorrel (*Rumex scutatus*), Curly dock (*Rumex crispus*).

Caution: avoid large amounts of sorrel if you have any stones, gout or gastric inflammation.

What kind of a weed is sorrel?

The *Rumex* genus of the knotweed family comprises docks, sorrels, knotweeds and knotgrasses. We focus on two abundant sorrels, common (*R. acetosa*) and sheep's (*R. acetosella*).

The names give the game away. *Rumex* is derived from Latin *rumo*, to suck; *acetosa* and *acetosella* from words for vinegar. In the unrelated wood sorrel (*Oxalis acetosella*), *oxis* is Greek for sour. Even 'vinegar' is from French *vin aigre*, fermented wine or acetic acid.

Sorrel leaves have been valued for this sourness as both food and medicine since prehistory.

Its success as a weed owed much to its wind-spread seeds, each plant yielding 2,000 or more; its roots can regrow from the smallest fragment. Not too fussy about soil quality, and with its sourness as a deterrent to grazing animals, it spread readily across continents.

Garden sorrel is the same species as common sorrel, but bred to have larger leaves. The wild plant has the advantage of being available for more of the year than its larger leaved garden counterpart. Another occasional British garden species is French, round-leaved or buckler-leaved sorrel (*R. scutatus*), so called because its leaves are shaped like a round shield or buckler.

If you are interested in foraging sorrel in your garden, in fields or pastures,

you should be aware that when young the leaves could be confused with a toxic common weed, lords and ladies or cuckoo pint (*Arum maculatum*), but the latter is a plant of shady places.

The pointed 'tails' or basal leaf lobes are the key thing to look for: in common sorrel the tails point backwards, looking as though, in forager John Rensten's words (2016), they have been 'cut by scissors' (see above); in sheep's sorrel, the tails point sideways or forwards; but in lords and ladies the tails are wholly rounded.

And to tell sorrel from the somewhat similar-looking docks, taste a leaf or fruit: sorrels are sharp and lemony, docks are sour and bitter.

The thing people know about sorrels is they contain oxalic acid. This gives the sour taste of sorrels but also underlies the various taste sensations of rhubarb and the vegetables spinach and chard.

In small quantities, such as normal food helpings, the effect is stimulating. The caution must be added, though, that taken in excess oxalic acid removes calcium from the blood, turning it to calcium oxalate, which might result in kidney stones. The same effect occurs if you eat rhubarb leaves.

But, we add straightaway, this arises only from wilful bingeing on sorrel; in forager John Wright's terms (2010), you must take a *sufficiently reckless dose*, eating it *by the bucketful*.

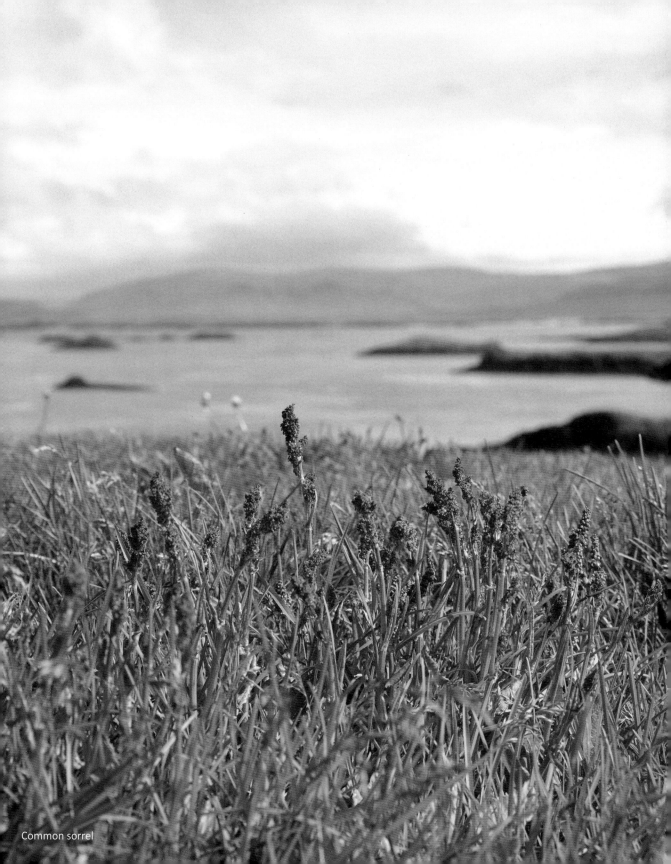
Common sorrel

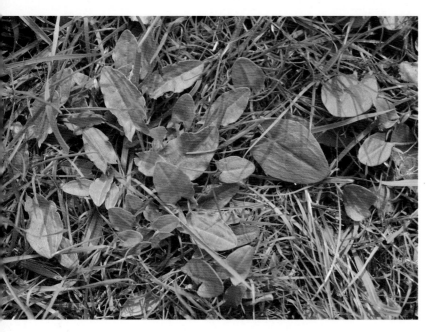

But the acidity message lingered: in 1699, John Evelyn called his book on salads *Acetaria: A Discourse of Sallets*.

Herbal & other uses of sorrel

Our ancestors knew that sorrel and lemons, with other sharp-tasting plants, were good against scurvy. We moderns say they contain high vitamin C, plus A and some B vitamins, as well as bioavailable minerals.

Mrs Grieve (1931) mentions 'conserva ligulae', a formerly made medicinal jam or conserve that combined wood sorrel leaves, sugar and orange peel. This went into a cooling drink for fever and scurvy patients.

Sorrel has long been used to curdle milk. Old posset recipes specified that spices were boiled in milk, and sorrel leaves added to the 'seething' mixture. In effect it was a plant rennet for making a green-colored cheese.

An old name for sorrel is greensauce. This also stood as a recipe name for a cold preparation of sorrel leaves pounded in a mortar with vinegar and sugar, and added to cold meats. Pease pudding and a green porridge were also derived from sorrel.

Herbally, sorrel is nutritive and stimulates digestion. It is cooling, anti-inflammatory (for stomach ulcers) and antioxidant. Once used to reduce fevers and infection, in northern climates it made a ready poultice for sores and bruises, and to reduce bleeding; the leaves were chewed for infected gums.

In Canada, sheep sorrel root and turkey rhubarb, another knotweed family member, formed part of the formulas for essiac and Ojibwa tea, with claimed anti-cancer properties.

In other uses, boiled sorrel leaves were used to remove stains from linen; in Iceland an infusion of the stems and leaves was used to polish silver and furniture. The roots could be boiled to yield an orange-red dye, the same color as the flower.

... [sorrel]: by nature cold, Abstersive, Acid, sharpning Appetite, asswages Heat, cools the Liver, strengthens the Heart; is an Antiscorbutic, resisting Putrefaction, and imparting so grateful a quickness to the rest, as supplies the want of Orange, Limon and other Omphacia, and therefore never to be excluded [i.e. from salads].
– Evelyn (1699)

Sorrel is much used in sauces both for the whole and the sick. It is a pleasant relish for the well, quickening up a dull stomach that is overloaded with everyday's plenty of dishes.
– Gerard (1597)

The Sorrel, or Green-sauce, is so common a plant in most meadows that few people are unfamiliar with its appearance, or with the pleasant acid taste of its leaves.
– Pierpoint Johnson (1862)

The history of sorrel

As a wild meadow plant, sorrel seeds occur in the European glacial record; in later times, including Bronze Age and Roman period Britain, the records are those of weeds linked with cultivation.

In Denmark both common and sheep's sorrel were found in the stomach contents of Tollund and Grauballe man, preserved from about 2,400 years ago.

But this is far more recent than the 8,000-year history of the related buckwheat (*Fagopyrum esculentum*), recorded in Tibet and west China. Buckwheat is gluten-free and used like a cereal (hence 'wheat').

Sorrel as a potherb, and wild-gathered, was the main source of sourness in European diets for many centuries; and in northern latitudes, too cold for citrus, was a rare source of vitamin C.

In the Middle Ages improved sorrel varieties were bred in France and Italy, notably the French sorrel. This arrived in England in the 16th century and gradually ousted the older commonly found species. Lemons too became more common items of the diet.

How to eat sorrel

The Victorian botanist Mrs Pratt (1866) declared what was then common knowledge: *Most persons have eaten [sorrel leaves] in childhood.* That was still true for Matthew a hundred years later, in his case being shown the more astringent wood sorrel (see box below).

It is still a buzz point in herb walks when you stoop down and pluck a sorrel leaf and offer it as a tasting. A nibble of sorrel is quite refreshing and thirst-quenching.

Its taste remains on cooking, provided you add the sorrel late on before serving. It will go a less attractive khaki brown color with heat, but you can add some more fresh leaves to restore the pleasing greenness, or combine sorrel with something like blanched nettle, which stays a vivid green.

Stainless steel cooking pans are best when cooking sorrel; aluminum ones can react with it to form an unwelcome toxin.

Traditional recipes include French sorrel soup, which is well known and rightly valued, and sorrel sauce, which is famed for fish. Dried sorrel leaves were mixed with sugar as a lemonade mix. Modern chefs make sorrel sorbet, perfect for cleansing the palate.

A reminder on quantity: the taste of sorrel is more a flavor enhancer than a meal in itself. Instinct tells us not to want too much sourness; we should heed the message.

Sorrel can be used wherever you need a little sharpness. It can replace lemon in zhug or in a tabbouleh salad. Try it simply whizzed up in some oil to sprinkle on roast potatoes.

Its [sorrel's] fresh, sappy sourness, when mixed with a little sugar, enhances both the sweetness and sourness of apples, making them taste amazingly fruity. Compare this with a plain apple fritter.
– Kapoor (2003)

Surelle. Take Surel, washe hit, grynde it [with a mortar and pestle], put a litle salt, therto, and strayne hit, and serue forth.
– Anon. (c1440)

The wider world of sorrels

Other plants with a sour, lemony taste are also referred to as sorrel.

The most common of these are the *Oxalis*, such as wood sorrel, *Oxalis acetosella.* Other species are often found as garden weeds, and vary in flavor from very lemony to quite mild. The clover-like leaves and the flowers make attractive additions to salad. If the three leaflets are pulled apart, they make perfect heart shapes, as on the right.

Tubers of *Oxalis tuberosa*, oca, are an important food crop in the Andes, and sometimes grown in gardens.

In South Africa another *Oxalis*, the yellow-flowered Cape sorrel or Bermuda buttercup, *Oxalis pes-caprae*, is enjoyed as a tart counter-taste to the sweet *waterblommetjies* stew and remains a popular potherb.

Jamaican sorrel or roselle is actually a hibiscus, *Hibiscus sabdariffa*, originally from West Africa. The red sepals and calyx are used to make a delicious sour drink.

The young leaves of curly or yellow dock, *Rumex crispus*, also taste similar to sorrel when cooked. Like sorrel, they immediately turn a khaki shade when heated, but they are very tasty. It is the only dock that tastes good, apart from its relative bistort, with its mild lemony taste, that is used in a spring 'dock' pudding.

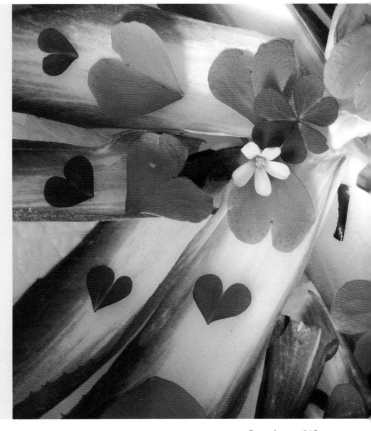

Sorrel Zhug

In this version of *zhug*, a spicy Yemeni sauce popular across the Middle East, we use sorrel in place of the traditional lemon juice. It's a very similar green sauce to *chermoula*. The recipe can be made as mild or hot as you like by adjusting the chillies used. The vibrant zingy flavor perks up sandwiches and goes well with a variety of cooked food or can be used as part of a mezze selection.

Use a small food processer or a stick blender for this. Add:
a handful of sorrel leaves
a handful of parsley leaves
two handfuls of coriander (cilantro) leaves
1 or 2 green chillies
1 clove garlic
pinch salt
pinch cardamom powder
enough extra virgin olive oil to make a smooth but thick purée

Taste and adjust as necessary.

Best used fresh, it will keep in the fridge for a few days, especially if covered with a thin layer of extra oil.

Alternatives: Sesame oil or hemp seed oil also work well in this recipe. Other weed greens such as chickweed and nipplewort can be used instead of parsley, but keep the coriander as the heart of the recipe.

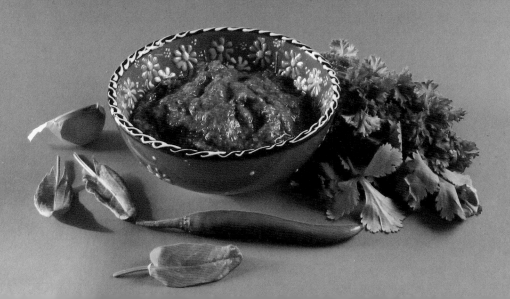

Sorrel **Pikelets**

These small oval pancakes are adapted from a recipe from Julie's Australian relatives, where pikelets are served cold with butter for afternoon tea. They can of course also be eaten warm with maple or other syrup.

Put in a bowl and stir to mix:
120g (1 cup) flour
1½ teaspoons baking powder
¼ teaspoon salt
2 teaspoons sugar
Add 120ml (1 cup) rice milk or almond milk
Add 2 tablespoons vegetable oil
1½ teaspoons golden syrup or maple syrup
2 tablespoons finely chopped sorrel leaves

The resulting batter should be medium thick. If you are using spelt flour it may be necessary to add another couple of tablespoons of flour.

Cook a tablespoonful at a time, in a lightly oiled cast iron skillet. Turn when the first side is full of bubble holes and is starting to set. They should be golden brown. Makes 15 to 20 pikelets.

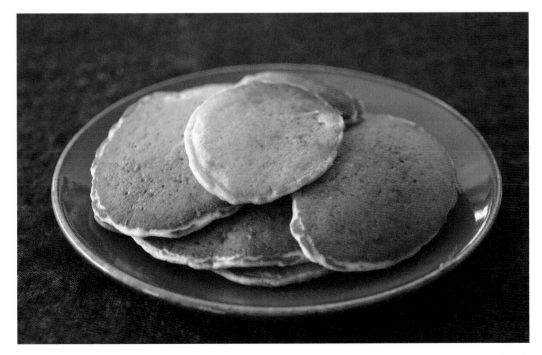

Sowthistle

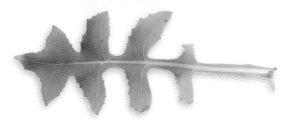

There are about 60 species of *Sonchus* or sowthistle found in temperate regions worldwide, often growing in arable fields, waste land and gardens. Sowthistles are enjoyed as food by many people around the world, but in other countries they are dismissed as invasive weeds. We think they are far too succulent to be restricted to pigs – we should eat them ourselves!

Asteraceae
Daisy family
(formerly Compositae)

Annuals, excepting perennial sow thistle.

Distinguishing features
• Sowthistles have hollow stems and a milky sap.
• Flower buds in all species are clustered on top of the flowering stem, unlike dandelions, which have one flower per stem and flatter leaves.
• The main species used as a food is **smooth sowthistle** (*Sonchus oleraceus*). It is an annual weed, like the other common species **prickly sowthistle** (*S. asper*). Both have smooth stems.
• The spininess of the leaves is an obvious distinction between the two, but the prickliness does vary considerably.
• Prickly sow thistle has shinier leaves.
• Smooth sowthistle has paler yellow flowers.
• In smooth sowthistle the basal lobes of the leaves spread out while in the prickly species the lobes are clasped to the stem.

Edible relatives: Perennial sowthistle (*S. arvensis*) is often much larger, the flowers are wider and rich yellow, and the flowering stems have sticky yellow hairs.

What kind of weed is sowthistle?
The sowthistles are members of the huge Aster family – with its more than 23,000 species – and are related to lettuce and dandelions, with which they share a milky sap.

As wild food they are enjoyed worldwide. One of them, smooth sowthistle, was given the accolade *oleraceus* (meaning tasty or potherb) by Linnaeus in 1753.

And it's not just human appreciation. Given the many country names for sowthistle that reference animals, this is evidently a favorite food in the farmyard and field.

Pigs do indeed seek it out (another name is sow bread), and it has been called dog's thistle, hare's lettuce and rabbit's meat (see box p224).

The other part of sowthistle's scientific name is *Sonchus*, or hollow (i.e. the stems). These stems contain a milky sap or latex, as do other wild Asters such as dandelion, wild lettuce and chicory. In each case the sap has been used as a worldwide home remedy for treating warts.

The name milk thistle, sometimes applied to *Sonchus* species, more correctly refers to the liver herb *Silybum marianum*, which features distinctive white veins across its spiny dark green leaves. It has purple flowers.

Writing in 1862, Pierpoint Johnson, a leading English botanical author,

aptly summarizes the twin poles of the human / sowthistle relationship: it is *a common and troublesome weed*, but also *an esculent vegetable, and … an exceedingly wholesome one*.

As a weed sowthistle is in a major league, being accounted a notifiable pest in 56 countries, earning it the designation (not meant kindly) of a cosmopolitan weed.

It is also classified as a ruderal, meaning a pioneer species that prospers on rough ground. In New Zealand it is among the first plant colonizts on lava fields once they cool.

The various *Sonchus* species are prolific in seed production, with Salisbury (1961) estimating that the largest specimens of smooth sowthistle could yield 40,000 seeds per plant, as against 60,000 for its prickly cousin and a much lower 13,000 for the perennial species.

Each of these seeds is equipped with its own parachute for onward wind-borne travel. The seeds are generally viable in the soil for at least 10 years and show potential high germination rates.

Perennial sowthistle has its own spreading mechanism in its prolific and tenacious underground stems, which earned it a country name of gutweed. Some of its roots can penetrate 3m (10ft) underground.

Another aspect of the unattractiveness of sowthistle to farmers is that the weeds can be host to several insect

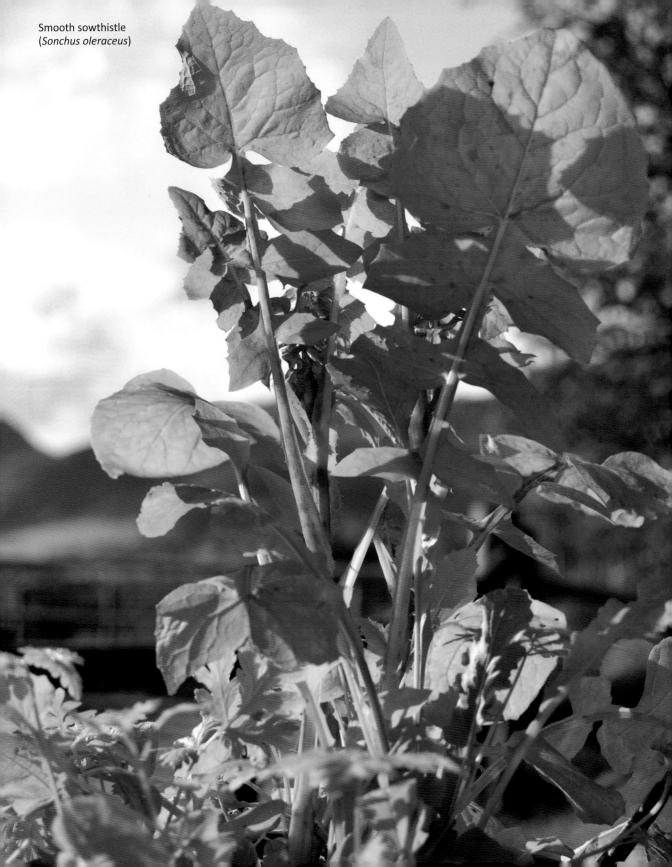

Smooth sowthistle
(*Sonchus oleraceus*)

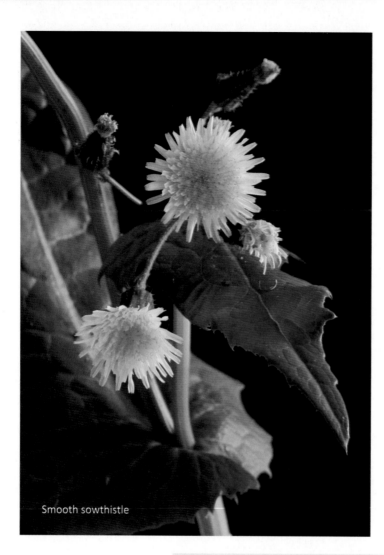

Smooth sowthistle

pests, such as leaf miners, lettuce root aphids and stem aphids.

Some aphids moreover can transmit LNYV, the lettuce necrotic yellow virus, and BYSV, the beet yellow stunt virus. Smooth sowthistle is known to be a host for the cotton bollworm, and has shown herbicide resistance, even to glyphosates.

In each case crop yields are reduced, sometimes by appreciable percentages.

In summary, notes CABI's Invasive Species Compendium, sowthistles are *almost perfect 'designer weeds'*.

The history of sowthistle

These are plants with a prehistory. Perennial sowthistle is recorded from several glacial and interglacial stages in the last half million years. The smooth and prickly species have oldest British datings of some 800,000 years ago for the smooth and over 400,000 years ago for the prickly.

In geographic origin *Sonchus* is thought to be Mediterranean, but spreading quickly worldwide once the ice caps retreated. There is little doubt it was a human food source from the outset, being quickly gathered, nutritious raw or cooked, and occurring wherever crops were grown.

The earliest western food record is probably that made in **Rome** by Pliny

[Smooth and prickly sowthistle are] *two of the world-conquering 'anthropophytes', plants that go around with man and flourish wherever he disturbs the soil.*

– Grigson (1955)

Flopsy bunny (and hare) food

Mrs Grieve's *A Modern Herbal* (1931) mentions that sowthistles are the nibble of choice for rabbits: there is no green food they devour more eagerly.

Rabbits also seek out other arable weeds we include in this book, such as dandelion, Jack by the hedge and cleavers.

In English folk history the plant was also known as hare's bush or even hare's palace. References to sowthistles and hares go back at least to the Pseudo-Apuleius, a 5th-century herbal by an unknown author: *if a hare eat of this herb [S. oleraceus] in summer when he is mad, he shall become whole.*

More than a thousand years later, the *Grete Herball* of 1526, the first illustrated printed herbal in English, explains why. Sowthistle was not only a food but a place of refuge for the hare: *if the hare come under it, he is sure that no beast can touch hym.*

the Elder (AD 23–79) in his *Naturalis Historia*. He recounts how the 'poor woman' Hecale gave the warrior Theseus a meal of sowthistle before he tackled the Bull of Marathon.

It has often been commented that the modern-day equivalent would be Popeye the Sailor Man and his can of spinach, powering him to defeat Bluto and rescue Olive Oyl.

Pliny pointed out that the plant was nourishing, curative and sustaining – he clearly thought it more a food than a weed.

The same was true in **China**, where an ancient saying went: *When the spring wind blows, sow thistles thrive. Wild plains turn into stores of food.* From the 7th century a more specific reference was made to Xiao Man, the season of late May: [In] *the days of Xiao Man are sow thistles at their best.*

Sowthistle, known in China as *kucai*, is still an important ingredient in Yunnan-style crispy red beans (*Suhongdou*).

In **Israel** sowthistle could be included in the Passover Seder Plate. The Talmud states that it is a duty for Jews to eat bitter plants (*maror*) on the first night of Passover, in memory of the bitterness of slavery in Egypt.

The chosen plants must be fresh and unsweetened. Other modern choices include romaine lettuce, chicory, horseradish or clover.

In **southern Africa** the Tswana in recent times gave sowthistle to their pigs when food was abundant and ate it themselves when it was not.

In fact sowthistle is one of the main potherbs of the area, known as *imifino* or *morogo*, the leaves and flowers being cooked as a spinach-like green with mielie meal (sweetcorn porridge). Other *imifino* plants include fat hen, dandelion and nettle.

Continuing this brief global look at sowthistle's history, Joseph Banks,

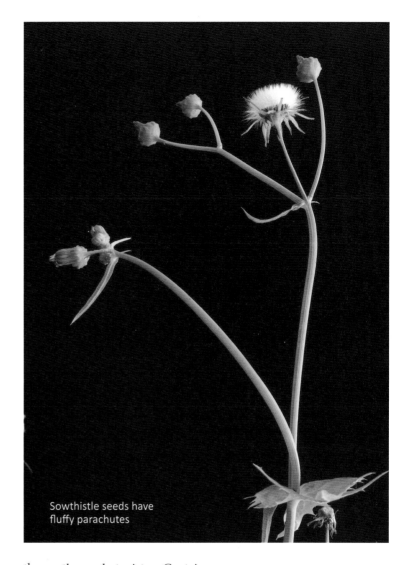

Sowthistle seeds have fluffy parachutes

the gentleman-botanist on Captain Cook's 1769–70 circumnavigation, saw sowthistle growing in Maori crops in **New Zealand**. The Maori called it *puwa* and considered it excellent food, as they still do.

Captain Cook was acutely aware of scurvy as a risk to his crew, and took advice that *puwa* (which included both smooth and prickly sowthistle) could be an effective answer for the problem, taking the medicine as a food. He insisted his crew make soup and salads using *puwa* but also the Brassica (cabbage family) species that came

Here's another 'weed,' despised by farmers and gardeners alike, that makes for wonderful eating. Sow thistle is a coarse, prickly, bitter green only fit for pigs – when it's mature. ... The [young] leaves taste so good after you sauté them with seasonings and complete the cooking in a sauce, you'll have an irresistible urge to pig out.

– Brill (2002)

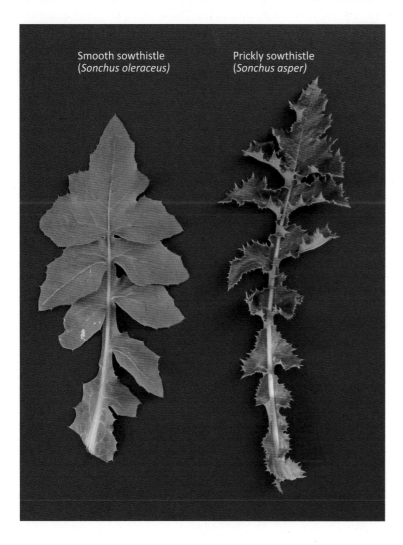

Smooth sowthistle
(*Sonchus oleraceus*)

Prickly sowthistle
(*Sonchus asper*)

as a face wash. For the Maori the latex made a good chewing gum.

Herbally, sowthistle is an underrated cooling bitter, less well known than dandelion but available at times when dandelion is not. Sowthistle poultices for bringing down fevers or applied to inflammatory conditions of the skin remain useful home remedies.

Another use for the plant dates from the early 20th century when Chinese residents of San Francisco claimed that sowthistle helped opium users break their addiction.

More recent research establishes that sowthistle is protective for the liver and kidneys through its polyphenol content. It acts as a strong free-radical scavenger, particularly against oxidative damage to the liver. This reflects earlier use as a hepatitis herb.

The diluted latex has been used experimentally to treat cough, asthma and bronchitis. This was known by John Parkinson, who wrote in 1640: *the milke that is taken from the stalkes when they are broken, given in drinke, is beneficial to those that are shortwinded and have a weesing withal.*

In modern China, sowthistle is a herb used by older men to maintain vitality and virility; it has been shown clinically to reverse erectile dysfunction. Gerard, writing in 1597, had another view: *The juice of these herbs doth cool and temper the heat of the fundament and privy parts.*

In New Zealand, the Maori preference for *puwa* may have protected them against colorectal cancers, clinical trials in 2002 found. Highly disadvantaged on most lifestyle indices, Maori who ate sowthistle and watercress had half the colorectal cancer incidence of the non-Maori population.

Whether the high levels of vitamin C and a range of bioavailable minerals in the plants were factors in these results requires further research.

... sowthistle springs up spontaneously in every spot which has been cultivated, and is generally used as a vegetable by the natives [i.e. the Maori].
– Taylor (1848)

... with their succulent crispness and refreshing hint of bitterness they [smooth sow thistle leaves] make a superb salad ...work fast as they quickly wilt – steep them in cool water until you need them.
– Mears & Hillman (2007)

to be known as Cook's scurvy grass (*Lepidium oleraceum*).

Only in the 20th century would it be proved that such vegetables, along with lime juice, were vitamin C-rich and that high C was the key to defeating scurvy.

In the Second World War New Zealanders on the home front were advised to collect *puwa* for its vitamins in the absence of imported oranges.

Herbal & other uses of sowthistle

We have noted the widespread popular use of sowthistle latex to treat warts, and it was also sometimes employed

How to eat sowthistle

Perennial sowthistle is best picked in the spring while the two annual species form rosettes over the winter and often have a second growth later on. Harvest them by cutting beneath the whole rosette or the flowering tops.

The young leaves and developing flower buds make the most succulent and pleasing eating.

Cut off the spines of prickly sowthistle with scissors before using. Bitterness is reduced in the cooking.

The stems themselves can be nibbled, rabbit style, after removing the tougher outer layer.

The young leaves and buds are eaten raw in salads worldwide, and in Italy quick boiling them in residual heat for less than 5 minutes, then adding olive oil and garlic, makes for a tender, easy meal. Substitute butter for olive oil if you prefer it.

The blogger Green Deane observes: *In southern Italy* Sonchus *invades crops there but they have the good sense to pick it and serve it with spaghetti.*

The Italian soup *minestrella* features sowthistle, while in Africa *ugaduagadu* is a vegetable cake made with sowthistle and cornmeal (mielie meal).

The stems, cut into circles of a centimeter or so, make a good pickle or can be candied.

Take care in picking your sowthistle as, unusually among the weeds in this book, it is prone to a powdery mildew. Leave infected plants alone.

You may think that sowthistle is a prosaic sort of weed, but you would be mistaken. In some cultures it is regarded as inhabiting a doorway to other worlds: in Italian fairy stories, reported William Fernie in 1897, the invocation 'open sow thistle' was used as English children would say 'open sesame'.

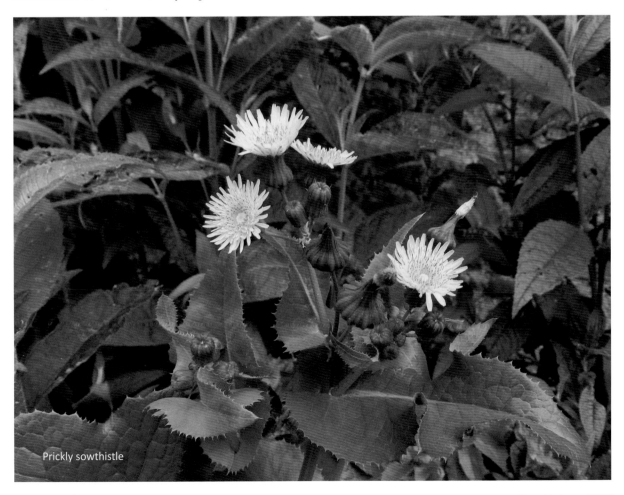

Prickly sowthistle

Simply Sowthistle

Sowthistle leaves are very tasty simply wilted and served with a little oil.

Pick a couple of handfuls of **sowthistle leaves** per person. If they are the prickly species, you'll need to trim the soft spines off the leaves with a pair of scissors. Smooth sowthistle needs no preparation.

Rinse the leaves and put in a pan over a gentle heat. Add **a little oil** if needed to prevent sticking, and stir until the leaves have wilted.

Alternatives: Stir-fry the wilted leaves in toasted sesame oil, and sprinkle with sesame seeds.

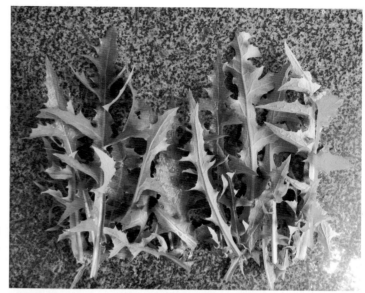

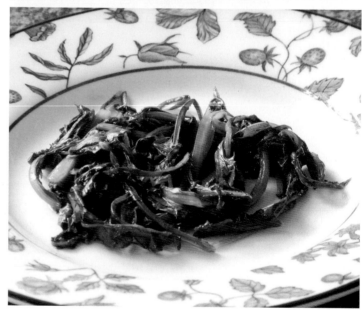

Sowthistle in **Peanut Sauce**

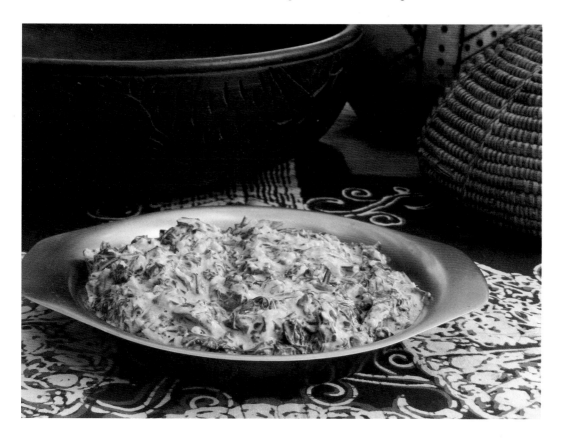

Begin with the picking: if you don't have enough sow thistle, combine with other greens such as fat hen, orache, nipplewort, swiss chard or spinach. Chop coarsely.

Heat **15ml (½ in) salted water** in a pan, then add **400g (14oz) sowthistle leaves** and cook until wilted. Drain, rinse in cold water.

Fry a finely chopped **shallot** in a little **toasted sesame oil**.

Blend **120ml (½ cup) coconut milk, juice of a lime, 1 or 2 cloves garlic, 2.5cm (1inch) piece fresh ginger** and **1 teaspoon chipotle paste**.

Use a stick blender to blend until smooth, then add the cooked shallots and **100g (⅓ cup) crunchy peanut butter**. Blend until mixed. Toss with the cooked greens. Serve warm or cold.

Alternatives: Fat hen, orache and nipplewort all work well in this recipe.

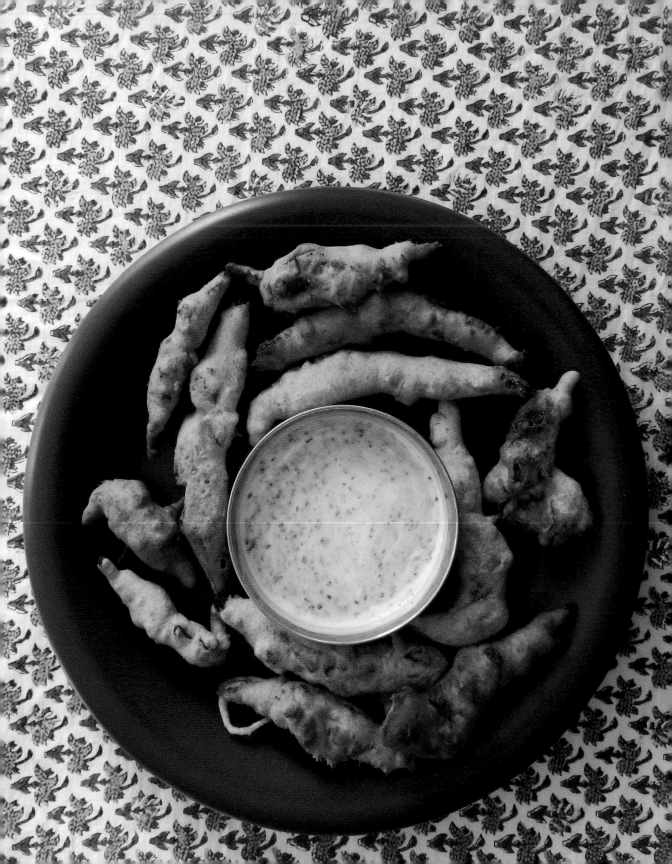

Sowthistle Bud Pakora

Sowthistle buds are succulent and delicious, and this is probably our favorite recipe for them.

Pick **sowthistle tops** when the flowers are still in bud. You'll probably be picking the top 7cm (3in) or so of the stalks, with the leaves surrounding the buds. Young flowers are fine but if any of the flowers have finished, just snip them off – once they start to go to seed, they become quite fibrous. Rinse well to remove any aphids that might be enjoying the buds.

In a small bowl, mix:
100g (1 cup) gram flour (or chickpea/garbanzo flour)
½ teaspoon turmeric powder
¼ teaspoon salt
¼ teaspoon paprika or chilli powder
¼ teaspoon coriander seed powder
125ml (½ cup) water

The mixture should be a thickish batter that will coat the sowthistle stems. Add more water if needed.

Deep fry a few at a time in hot **vegetable oil**, turning over with a slotted spoon so that both sides cook evenly. Cook until golden, then put on a plate covered with kitchen roll (paper towel).

Serve with your favorite sauce or chutney to dip. Try mixing a little gremolata (see p199) with coconut yogurt or oat cream, or use a coconut and lime chutney.

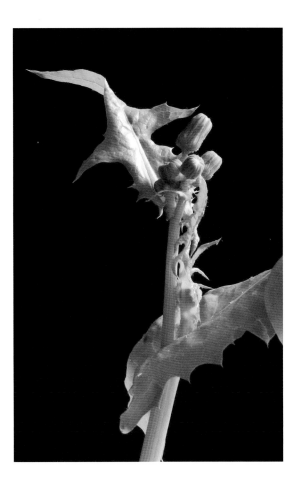

Sowthistle with Noodles

This simple dish brings oriental flavors to complement sowthistle. A choice of noodles lets you vary the recipe. We used **sen lek** wholemeal noodles, but buckwheat noodles or rice noodles also work well.

Put about **200g (7oz) of noodles** on to cook in **boiling salted water** according to the package directions.

While the noodles cook, stir fry **a couple of handfuls of sowthistle leaves** in **toasted sesame oil** in a wok. Add some **minced garlic** and **finely grated fresh ginger**. If you like your noodles spicy, add some **chilli flakes**.

When the noodles are cooked, drain them and rinse briefly in **cold water**. Add them to the wok and stir to mix all the ingredients. Taste, and add **more toasted sesame oil** and **tamari soy sauce to taste**.

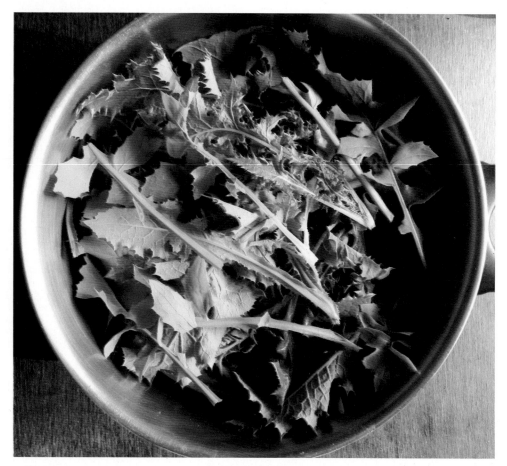

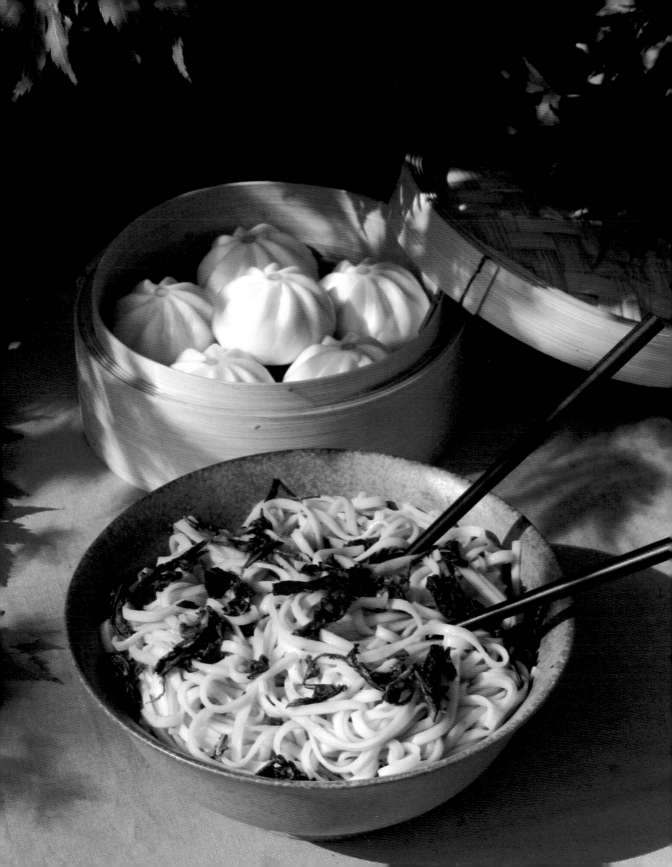

Sowthistle & Corn **Muffins**

Sowthistle leaves are a tasty addition to these slightly spicy muffins, which are a bit like mini corn breads. They are great for breakfast or served with beans, and are both vegan and gluten-free.

Makes 12 muffins.

If you have a food processor, you can mix everything in there – easy! But if you don't, simply chop the corn kernels, then mix everything in a bowl.

Preheat the oven to 200C/400F. Lightly grease a muffin tray.

Mix together:
100g (1 cup) sweetcorn/corn kernels, roughly chopped
30g (1 cup) chopped sowthistle leaves
170g (1 cup) medium polenta/corn meal
100g (1 cup) gram flour (or chickpea/garbanzo flour)
250ml (1 cup) water
60ml (¼ cup) oil
1 or 2 chillies, chopped finely
1 clove of garlic, minced (or ½ teaspoon garlic powder)
2 teaspoons baking powder
½ teaspoon salt

Spoon the resulting batter evenly into the oiled muffin tins.

Bake for 20 minutes, until the tops go slightly golden and an inserted skewer comes out clean.

Cool in the pan for a few minutes, then tip the muffins out.

Serve warm.

They can be stored for a few days in an airtight container in the fridge, but are best if warmed through before serving.

Alternatives: Sprinkle the tops of the muffins with Jack by the hedge seed, sesame seeds or nigella seed before baking.

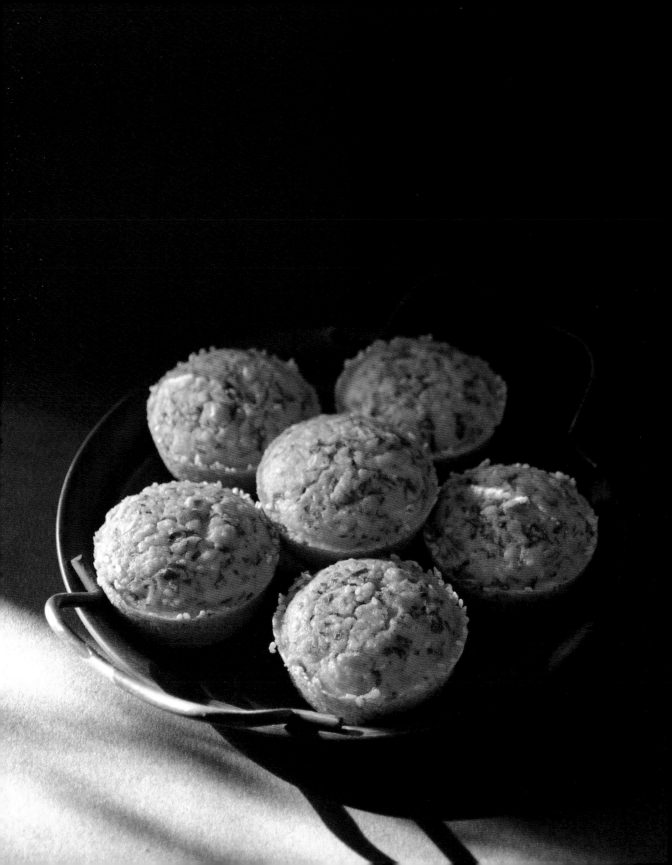

Spear Thistle

This familiar prickly meadow weed with its ferocious spines does not look edible at all, but those spines are there to protect it from being eaten by browsing animals precisely because it is nutritious. Spear or bull thistle *(Cirsium vulgaris)*, the chosen species here, does not employ bitterness or latex in the stem as an additional deterrent; once disarmed it is sweet and tasty. We recommend our favorite, easy-to-make 'thistle-ade'. Presenting it to guests makes good theatre as well as offering a surprisingly nourishing drink.

Asteraceae
Daisy family
(formerly Compositae)

Biennial.

Edible parts: Leaves, year round; root, autumn and spring; stalk, late spring; flowers, summer.

Distinguishing features: The spininess of thistles makes them unmistakable. Spear (bull) thistle is a common weed in gardens, fields and grazing land, and as its name suggests is formidably spiny. In its first year the plant grows as a rosette of leaves. When it flowers in its second year, it can reach 1.5m (5ft) or more tall, and is topped with magenta flowers protected by spiny bracts. The seeds have a plume of feathery hairs – thistledown – which drifts them away on the wind.

Edible relatives: All thistles are edible. Artichoke (*Cynara scolymus*) and cardoon (*C. cardunculus*) are grown for their flower buds and edible stalks respectively. Cabbage thistle (*Cirsium oleraceum*) is also sometimes cultivated.

What kind of a weed is spear thistle?

Thistles have always had a bad rep. The first plants to be named in the Bible are thorns and thistles, described in Genesis as growing on 'cursed ground'.

Shakespeare repeats the accusation in *King Henry V* where the Duke of Burgundy laments a war-ravaged France in which *nothing teems but hateful docks, rough thistles, kecksies* [cow parsley], *burs* [burdock], *losing both beauty and utility*.

The Authorized Version quoted above is dated 1611 and Shakespeare's play is about 1599. They display a similar worldview, which still persists, about waste land and its wild or weedy plants. But what does a field of purple-headed spear thistles really tell us?

Thistles are very often a plant of overgrazed pastures, and they are there on a mission of phytoremediation. If you haven't come across the term before, it applies to plants that detoxify, decontaminate and regenerate poisoned, polluted or exhausted land.

So a thistle field is one that has been badly farmed – 'cursed' indeed – and is being healed. The problem is with the farming practice, not the weeds.

Yet the UK Weed Act 1959 names as 'injurious' five land-healing species – spear (bull) and creeping thistle, curly and broad-leaved dock, and ragwort (the latter poisonous to mammals).

Each is a sturdy, persistent and abundant pioneer, and what they are doing ecologically is making farming-abused or brownfield land fit for later plants and ultimately trees to flourish.

But this natural succession process takes some years, and these highly visible weeds damage today's profits by lowering crop yields.

The current UK government advice on environmental management still talks of 'infestation' by the five criminalized weeds. The authorities remain uneasy with wildness and untidiness.

In other parts of the world thistles are 'notifiable' or 'aliens' that outcompete native plants agriculturally and in natural environments, and hence must be destroyed, usually by glyphosates.

Spear or bull thistle (*Cirsium vulgaris*) is a biennial with formidable distribution capacity via its seed parachutes, and is particularly invasive in subsaharan Africa, Australia and Japan.

Another common species, the perennial creeping, Canada or California thistle (*C. arvense*), with its pale purple pompom of a flower, has deep taproots and horizontal underground runners.

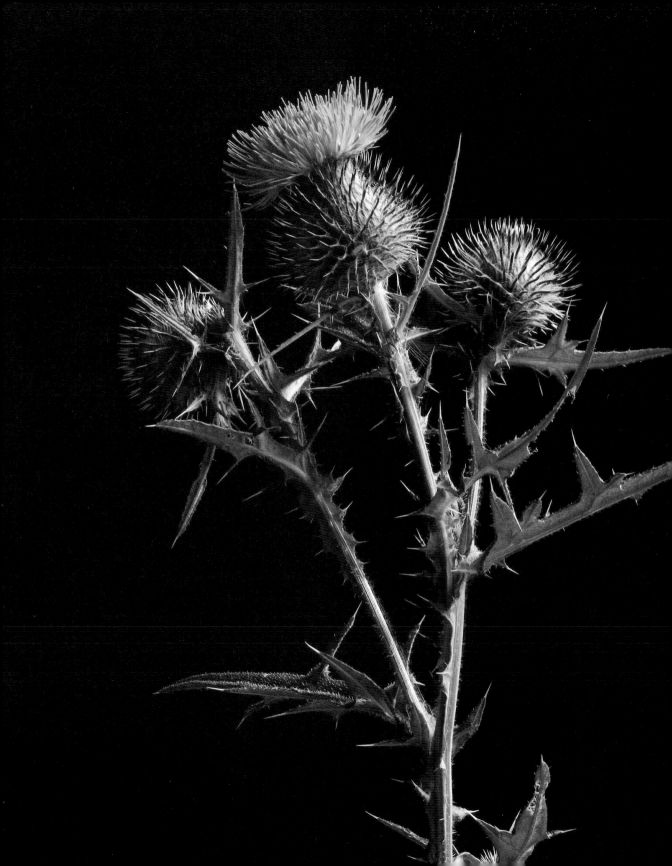

Her brittle runners emerge above ground as clonal plants, and moreover any single piece of them left by ploughing will regenerate into a new plant.

Invasive in northern states of the US and New Zealand, the presence of *C. arvense* caused lost revenue of about NZ$700 million [some £400m] on the latter country's farms in 2016.

The history of thistles

Thistle is symbolic of Scotland, whose highest civilian honor is the Order of the Thistle, with the appropriate motto 'nobody attacks me with impunity'.

You might imagine that thistles are classified by their degree of spininess. But there are non-spiny thistles, like the Scottish resident known as melancholy thistle (*Cirsium heterophyllum*). It is soft and pretty rather than a formidable warrior like its spear thistle cousin.

The main forms into which thistles have evolved concern rather the degree of latex found in the stems.

The Cardueae subgroup has none. In this group are spear and creeping thistle, burdock, milk thistle (*Silybum marianum*), cotton thistle (*Onopordum acanthium*) – actually the real 'Scotch thistle' – and globe artichoke.

The other subgroup of true thistles is the Lactuceae, which do have stem latex. Typical species are chicory, lettuces, nipplewort, sowthistles and dandelions.

Spines and latex are both forms of self-defence, with the intention of making the thistles unpalatable and off-putting to animal browsers.

As forager Miles Irving points out (2009), with such weapons at hand the plants do not need additional bitterness or toxicity as a deterrent.

A spear thistle rosette in winter

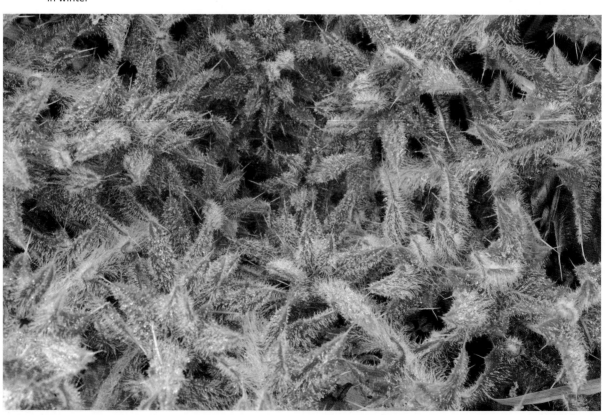

Both subgroups include plants that have been transformed from wild weed to cultivated food, and the history of thistles could equally be seen as this process of taking advantage of their potential esculency (edibility).

Herbal & other uses of thistles

Sir Edward Salisbury (1961) describes taproots of creeping thistles in black Russian soils growing 18 feet (5.5m) down, with a single plant capable of spreading radially 20–40 feet (6–12m) in the growing season.

These are exceptional, but he finds it *one of worst pasture weeds, and this despite the fact that it is so often sterile.*

Yet the converse also holds: these deep roots bring up far-down nutrients and make them available to nearby plants. Australian ecologists have observed that in a thistle meadow, adjacent grasses and other plants grow better for the connection.

The deep roots also aerate soil compacted from overgrazing and help to minimize topsoil loss from the wind.

Thistles also have wildlife benefits. Thistledown is a food prized by goldfinches, the flowers provide nectar for bees, and spear thistle leaves are the food plant of painted lady butterflies.

Thistles can also make excellent fodder for cattle and horses if sufficiently crushed to disarm the spines.

Then there is the area of medicinal benefit from the thistle family. Summarizing, most species are kidney- and liver-protective and bile-supporting, especially milk thistle, which has a role in treating liver damage induced by chemotherapy and is a well-known (if not particularly effective) hangover remedy.

The thistles in effect act on the liver as they can do on the land by removing toxins and stimulating cell growth; taken as a tea they will do something similar for relieving headaches.

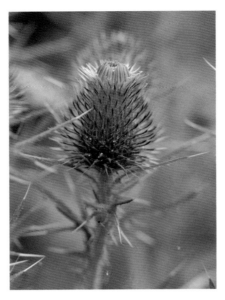

The purple part of the flower can be pulled out and chewed like gum

How to eat thistles

There are no poisonous thistles and all are edible to some degree. Our particular favorite is a spear thistle leaf alkalizing drink (see p241), though the stems, stalks, roots and flowers all have edible potential.

The key is to follow the plant's life cycle and be alert to the spines as you harvest and cook.

Take the spear thistle. As a biennial it germinates over summer and builds up a basal rosette of leaves and tap root to survive its first winter. Next spring and summer the tall stems (sometimes 2m or 6ft 6in high) grow quickly, with large lateral spiny leaves and the purple-red 'shaving brush' flower and seed head following. After the seeds parachute away, the plant dies.

The time to dig up the roots and basal leaves is in the first winter and the next spring before all that stored energy goes into stem and leaf formation.

The time to savor the juicy inner stems is in the second growing season (early summer) before the flowers appear; at that stage the stems turn woody and rigid to support what has become a tall, structural plant.

The young shoot for leaves [of milk thistle] *in the spring, cut close to the root, with part of the stalk on, is one of the best boiling sallads that is eaten, and surpasses the finest Cabbage.*
– Bryant (1783)

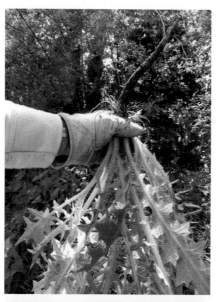

Spear thistle stem harvesting requires stout gloves until the spines have been removed

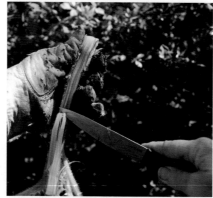

Thistle stalks are a great source of mineralized, ... highly alkalized water, ... alive with the brilliance of the thistle plant. ... Thistle offers the body a true alkaline experience.
– Blair (2014)

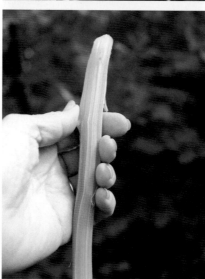

So, come May, try spear thistle **stems** as a foraged raw snack while walking. Wearing stout gloves, test the springiness of the stem: if it is flexible it is ready to harvest.

Using your sharp foraging knife, cut off a stem at the base. Hold the stem upside down (there are few spines at the base anyway) and chop off the leaves.

Next scrape away the spines and outer skin layer of the stem. You have a stick of succulent inner thistle pith that tastes celery-like (some people get cucumber), alkaline and refreshing.

Otherwise boil these stripped stems as a soup or in a stew, or fry them with miso. Alternatively, try pickling them by boiling them and maturing in vinegar. Milk thistle stems are said to be more tasty than any cabbage, making what Bryant (1783) called a 'boiling sallad' (quote p239).

In southern Europe **cardoons**, a thistle relative and originator of cultivated artichoke, are bred for their tasty stalks. In Spain they are often blanched by burying them underground before harvest.

If **rosette leaves** picked (with gloves) for boiling turn out to be too bitter for your taste, try double-boiling them by replacing your first water with a fresh lot and reheating. When cooking rosette leaves, ensure you remove all spines as boiling will not soften them.

The **flowerhead** has an edible heart if you have the patience to free it of its armour. The purplish stamens should not be discarded as they make excellent chewing gum. The 'leaves' of **globe artichoke** are actually sepals enveloping its flowerhead.

Roots of spear thistle are best dug up in winter or the following spring, but remember you need the landowner's permission to harvest any roots. If you can, use plants growing on your own land. Creeping thistle roots are best in autumn, swollen by a summer of active growth.

Cleaned and chopped up, the roots can be steamed or roasted, as our forefathers did. **Salsify** is a thistle relative eaten for its black-skinned roots.

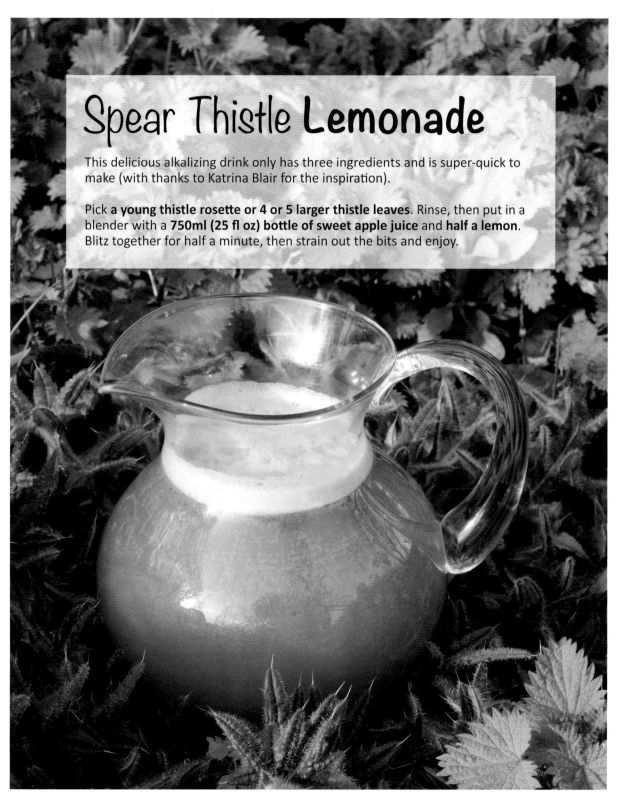

Spear Thistle **Lemonade**

This delicious alkalizing drink only has three ingredients and is super-quick to make (with thanks to Katrina Blair for the inspiration).

Pick **a young thistle rosette or 4 or 5 larger thistle leaves**. Rinse, then put in a blender with a **750ml (25 fl oz) bottle of sweet apple juice** and **half a lemon**. Blitz together for half a minute, then strain out the bits and enjoy.

Yarrow

Yarrow (*Achillea millefolium*) is a major medicinal herb, an abundant garden flower, with cultivars in almost every color, and a weed that some gardeners find troublesome. It has an ancient provenance, far earlier than the battlefields of Troy where it is usually first referenced, and we make use of its flavor in an adapted Turkish mezze recipe as well as an original Za'atar mixed with ground ivy.

Asteraceae (formerly Compositae) Daisy family

Perennial.

Edible parts: Mainly leaves, also flowerheads and young stalks.

Distinguishing features: The combination of feathery, deeply cut, dark green leaves and a flattish flowerhead of dull white or pink individual florets is distinctive. The smell is slightly aromatic when the leaves are crushed.

But be aware that yarrow can misdirect: the flowerhead is umbel-shaped but yarrow is not an Apiaceae or even related; the leaves appear to be manifold (the species name *millefolium* means thousands of leaves) but are a relatively small number so finely dissected as to look multiform.

Caution: Yarrow contains trace amounts of thujone and camphor, which on extended and heavy ingestion could build up toxicity. Yarrow can sometimes cause skin allergies to those sensitive to Asteraceae family species. Medicinal doses are not recommended for pregnant or breast-feeding women, or for infants.

What kind of a weed is yarrow?

Yarrow (*Achillea millefolium*) is a familiar garden perennial and weed of borders and lawns. It has persistent and quick-growing but not very deep underground rhizomes. These develop into tangled knots that can squeeze out neighboring plants, giving rise to small yarrow colonies.

Yarrow's other means of spreading is through small, almost transparent seeds. These are light and can be carried on the wind but more usually drop beneath the parent plant when ripe. Again this adds to the colonial habit of yarrow that can annoy gardeners.

On the other hand, some gardeners welcome yarrow as a companion plant, one that assists neighboring plants by loosening up compacted soil.

Biodynamic gardeners esteem yarrow as one of six constituents of a standard compost (with chamomile, nettle, oak, dandelion and valerian). Minute amounts of these help in soil decomposition and humus formation; yarrow specifically promotes transfer of potassium and sulphur to plant roots.

But if removal of yarrow is the goal, control is relatively straightforward, by hoeing or slicing the plants with a spade. The roots can readily be pulled out manually, but any dormant root buds that break off will produce daughter plants.

Sir Edward Salisbury (1961) states that yarrow plants typically have some 3,000 seeds along with a high rate of germination (75%).

Subsequent research has increased the probable number of seeds per plant and adds that yarrow's dormancy periods are relatively long.

It is also able to withstand drought and grows in most soil types, except those that are wet or over-acidic.

Such factors make yarrow a successful wild colonizer, but also a weed where humans do not want it.

Its native origin is not known, but that is unsurprising given its antiquity (see next section). Probably beginning in Eurasia, it has thrived in temperate climates, is a good self-spreader and has been well distributed by human colonizers north and south as both an ornamental and medicinal plant.

The consensus is that it arrived in North America after the retreat of the ice caps, or in the previous interglacial period. It was and is still widely used by First Peoples. European settlers from the late sixteenth century onwards added their own yarrow species.

The garden writer Ken Thompson (2009) takes a perceived unwelcome presence of yarrow to its logical conclusion: if you really cannot eliminate it, or allow it as ground cover, embrace it and create a yarrow lawn.

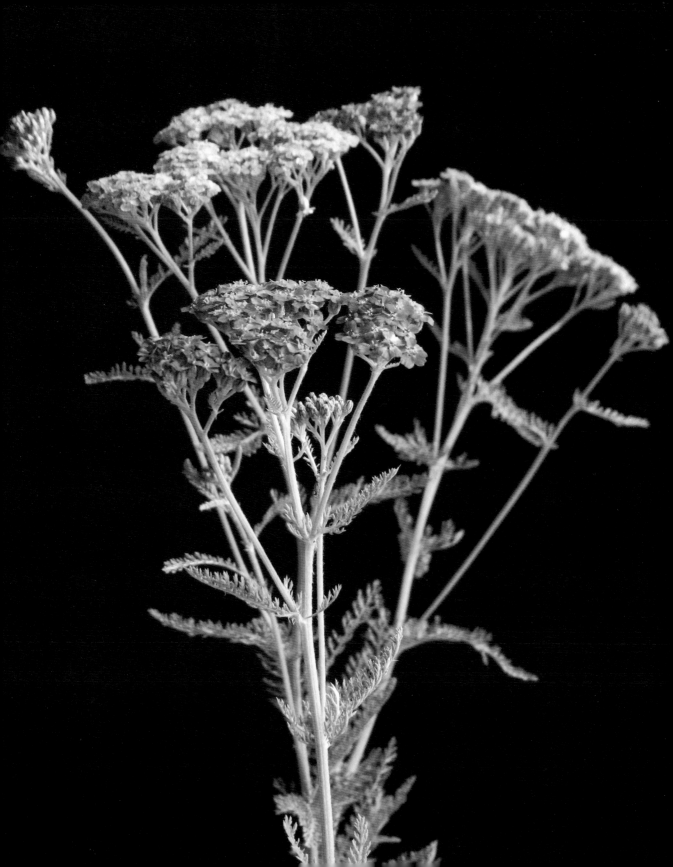

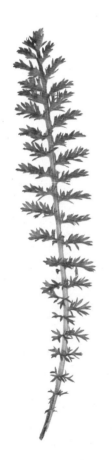

Yarrow is close to chamomile in botanical classification, and makes a pleasant alternative to it in lawns. Both are fragrant, and yarrow has perhaps the prettier white or pink flowers; both make wonderful teas and herbal preparations.

But this proposal will not be appreciated in Australia and New Zealand, where yarrow was introduced, perhaps in fodder, as an ornamental or for medicinal qualities.

In the Snowy Mountains of Australia it has proliferated in tourist areas, along newly created roads and visitor buildings, and outcompetes native subalpine and alpine floras. It is a major weed of mixed crop areas in parts of New Zealand.

It is also termed an agricultural invasive in Argentina and Chile, but lacks this reputation in northern temperate zones.

The history of yarrow

The story of yarrow usually starts with Achilles and the Trojan War, over 3,000 years ago. We want to begin much further back, some 50,000 years ago, where there is hard evidence for yarrow's links to our ancestors.

An archaeological cave site called El Sidrón in Asturias, northern Spain, uncovered in 1994, yielded up to 13 Neanderthal skeletons. One had analyzable dental calculus or tartar.

Scientists identified yarrow and German chamomile (*Matricara chamomilla*) remains within the tartar, and suggested that the presence of these close Asteraceae relatives, both bitter healing herbs, indicates medicinal more than food use.

Remarkably, the El Sidrón tooth samples had the TAS2R39 gene, a marker for bitterness. This has been interpreted as meaning the Neanderthals avoided toxic plants but favored bitter ones in efforts to control internal parasite or bacterial infection.

This is a very early, if not the earliest, marker of herbal use anywhere by ancestral humans or Neanderthals.

Another Neanderthal cave site, Shanidar, in Iran, from a similar date, had pollen remains that included yarrow, grape hyacinth and hollyhock. The flowers had been placed on a grave with an intact skeleton.

The predominant interpretation is that the flowers were left as a sign of mourning for a family member, although a counter-proposal is that local wild rodents (in this case gerbils) had used the cave to store plant material.

Our own opinion is that Neanderthals, alongside humans at the same period, were master herbalists who needed to know which plants were medicinal or good to eat and which should be avoided. Such survival knowledge parallels the emotional intelligence to love and mourn a family member (see Shipley & Kindscher 2016).

Coming forward in time, the antiquity of herbal and food use for yarrow is patchily confirmed by archaeology and later in written accounts in the Fertile Crescent, Egypt, China, India and through to classical Greece and Rome.

This brings us to Achilles and his fabled use of yarrow. We are told he was taught medicine by the centaur Chiron, became a Spartan general and saw to the supply of yarrow leaves as a wound herb on the battlefields of Troy, in modern Turkey.

This virtuous tale arose in folk stories but, interestingly, was not later confirmed in Greek and Roman authors, from Homer onwards. Archaeology so far has not shown the presence of a yarrow species in Turkey at that time.

Sustainable origin myth or not, herbally the Achilles story does make good sense. Supreme as a blood stauncher, yarrow leaves packed in a wound dramatically stop bleeding, while the plant's antimicrobial and antibacterial qualities keep the wound clean.

Yarrow as a first aid panacea has relieved battle wounds and saved lives in many wars, even 1914–18. Accordingly it accumulated military names like soldier's woundwort, staunchweed and herbe militaris.

But, with a mordant irony worthy of the gods, yarrow could not prevent the death by bleeding of its name-giver. Even semi-gods had to have their weak point, known universally as the Achilles heel since the day Paris shot a poison arrow into the one part of his body where Achilles was mortal.

Some accounts say it was Apollo, god of healing, but also of archery, who guided the arrow. He had good reason as Achilles had killed two of his sons and then Apollo's favorite, Hector.

Returning from 'wounded warrior' myth to yarrow the herb, it was one of the nine sacred plants of the Anglo-Saxons – interestingly, again alongside chamomile. It was given the common name of yarrow at about this time.

Commercially, it has never been a major herb crop but is largely supplied from fields in southeastern and eastern Europe.

Herbal & other uses of yarrow

The term panacea, or cure-all, is frequently applied to yarrow. It is recorded in the Native American ethnobotany database (NAEB) 374 times for specific applications (2003) – a huge spread. It is in fact one of the most used herbal medicines in the world.

... the iodine of the meadows and fields.
– Mességué (1979)

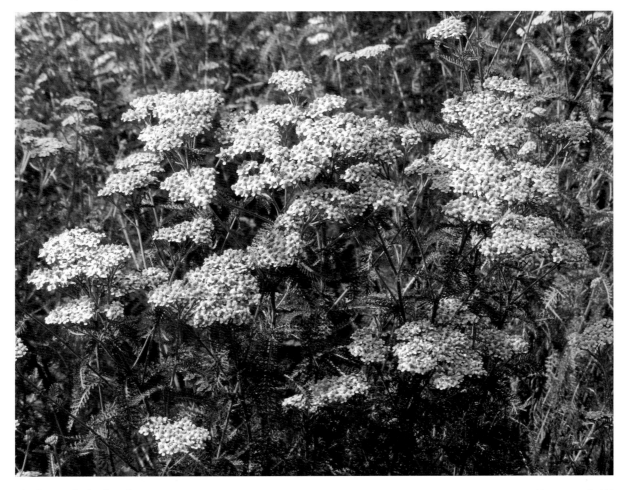

Yet being a wound herb is no longer yarrow's defining characteristic. Clearly, the level of everyday wounding is far less than in previous eras, and rather than battlefields we have kitchens, gardens, stairs and other sites of domestic jeopardy.

The *British Herbal Pharmacopoeia* (1996), for example, describes yarrow as 'official' as a diaphoretic (sweat-inducer in treating fevers). Commission E, the equivalent regulatory body in Germany, recommends yarrow for loss of appetite and mild dyspepsia.

In our household, however, yarrow remains foremost a first aid blood herb. We let self-planted wild yarrow flourish in cracks in the flagstones within a few yards of the kitchen door, and use it often.

When Matthew once had a nosebleed he first sought some cotton balls. Bad move, as he found: withdrawing the cotton balls only restarted the bleeding. But a spit poultice of yarrow leaves, that is, a few leaves chewed for ten seconds or so and put into the nostrils, stopped the blood, with no harm done.

In another incident our young adult son's friend didn't duck under a low beam in our house and gashed his scalp. Julie ran out into the garden

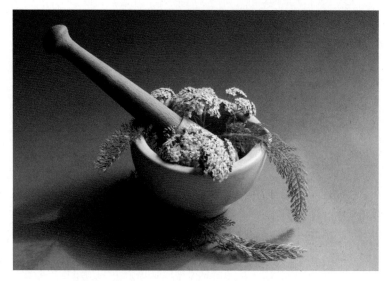

for the yarrow and packed the raw, bleeding wound, soon bringing the blood flow to a halt.

Then Julie's friend, who happened to be present, made her own contribution to the healing. She asked the injured party if she could plait his own long hair across the wound. He agreed, and the braid over the yarrow held the wound closed like stitches would.

After a few minutes the poor victim, groggy from blood loss and shock, but otherwise fine, could function again, with a lesson learned about low beams.

American herbalist Matthew Wood (2009) calls yarrow *master of the blood*, a haemostatic or normalizer of blood function. It can clot or unclot blood as the situation demands, regulating blood flow by thickening or thinning, and is known to reduce blood pressure.

This mechanism partly explains yarrow's effectiveness in hemorrhages, caused by wounds or excessive menstruation, rectal bleeding from hemorrhoids or bloody urine, when there is bright red blood.

Improved blood circulation at the extremities is also an aspect of another strong action by yarrow as a fever herb.

Causing therapeutic sweating, yarrow was sometimes called 'Englishman's quinine', especially in treating ague, a once-prevalent form of malaria. A hot tea from dried or fresh leaves, sometimes with elderflowers or peppermint, was used in breaking fevers, for common cold and flu, throat inflammations and lung conditions.

Yarrow's astringency can help relieve diarrhea and mild stomach discomfort. It is an appetite enhancer and supports the liver and gall bladder.

Yarrow's many other herbal and associated uses include:

• A tobacco substitute and snuff; in 1800 the herbal campaigner Richard Brook wrote: *To those who wish to smoke untaxed tobacco, the dried leaves of yarrow will be found one of the best English substitutes.* Sneezewort, a close relative of yarrow, was given its name for its use as a snuff in Scotland.

• A liqueur called Iva is made from *A. moschata*, the diminutive Swiss yarrow.

• In Sweden yarrow was called field hops for its use in brewing. The great botanical classifier Linnaeus held that beer brewed with yarrow was more intoxicating than that from hops.

• Yarrow stalks are used in telling the I Ching, the classic Chinese method of divination.

• In Iran yarrow is a natural yellow dye for carpets.

• In the American north yarrow smoke is a mosquito repellent, and yarrow stalks are smouldered as smudges to purify a space.

• Yarrow tea in baths is an herbal soak or steam for facials. As a lotion for the scalp it is said to help in restoring hair.

• It has an anodyne action on stomach cramps, arthritis, rheumatism and in relieving toothache or earache.

Use fresh or dried yarrow leaves or flowerheads as a tea, soaking in boiled water for about 5 minutes. The dried form is more bitter and medicinal.

Here are two yarrow-related extracts from our July tasting diary one year:

Today (22.7) we tried equal parts fresh fennel and yarrow tea, brewed for 5 minutes. The fennel makes it bright yellow. The bitterness of the yarrow is nicely balanced by the sweetness of the fennel. Tasty, mellow. Thanks to John Rensten [2016] for a good recipe.

Today (23.7) Julie made morning tea with yarrow and mint. Smooth, and the yarrow did enhance the mintiness of the other ingredient. It's a good mixer!

Distilled yarrow water is a beautiful blue color and is wonderful as a digestive aid.

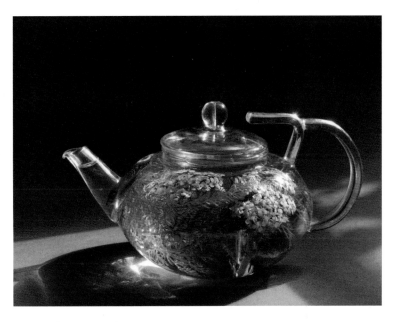

How to harvest and eat yarrow

Yarrow is easy to gather, the leaves stripping readily from the stems, particularly when dry; the flowerheads and stalks are tough, and scissors or secateurs are needed. Avoid picking plants located very close to roads.

For drying, gather whole stalks, bind them at the base with twine or string, and hang them upside down inside a paper bag. If you have one, use a dehydrator. Your dried yarrow should last a few months, and at least long enough for sweet new growth to reappear in the garden.

Dried yarrow is more bitter than the fresh herb, so keep this in mind when cooking with yarrow.

It makes a good vinegar or oxymel (vinegar with honey added) and a salad dressing – adding lemon and sugar helps draw out its flavor.

The Danish restaurant Noma features yarrow flowers in its green butter recipe, and yarrow is part of its trademark 'weeds on a plate'.

Weeds recipe-maker Vivien Weise (2004) suggests a baked yarrow polenta topped by sautéed almonds.

[yarrow tea is] amazingly good. … Why this tea ever went out of fashion is a mystery to me.

– Phillips (1983)

Dried and crushed they [yarrow flowers] make a fantastic addition to any za'atar or bouquet garni. You wouldn't believe how how strongly just one tiny flower can taste!

– Wilde (2019)

Yarrow Za'atar

Za'atar or zatar is the name for *Origanum syriacum* or *Satureja thymbra*, aromatic herbs that grow through the Mediterranean to the Middle East. It is also the name of a herb blend with these plants or a herb mix usually made up of dried thyme, oregano, marjoram, sumac, toasted sesame seeds, and salt.

As with any ancient recipe, there are many variations and opinions on how it should be made, so we felt free to create our own version with local weeds, taking inspiration from our friend and fellow forager Monica Wilde.

For the dried herbs, crumble the yarrow leaves and break the florets apart, discarding stems and stalks. Toast sesame seeds by dry frying in a pan with no oil until they are aromatic and light brown – shake or stir frequently to brown them fairly evenly.

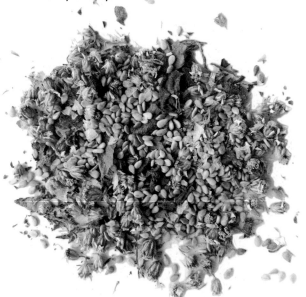

Mix roughly equal parts by volume of:
dried yarrow flowers and leaves
dried ground ivy leaves
toasted sesame seeds

and add **salt flakes** and **dried sorrel to taste**.

Serve with pita bread to dip in olive oil and then the za'atar mix, or use as a seasoning to add at the end of cooking various savory dishes.

Yarrow Mercimek Köftesi

This is a popular mezze dish in Turkish cuisine, made here with fresh yarrow leaves instead of the usual parsley.

Rinse **150g (¾ cup) red lentils** until the water runs clear. Put them in a saucepan with **400ml (1¾ cups) water** and bring to a boil, then reduce the heat, cover and simmer for 15 minutes.

Remove the pan from the heat and add **150g (¾ cup) bulghur**. Cover again and let stand for 15 minutes to allow the bulghur to swell.

In another pan, fry **a diced onion in 60ml (¼ cup) olive oil** for 5 minutes, then add **1 tablespoon tomato paste, ½ tablespoon salt, 1 teaspoon cumin powder** and **½ teaspoon chilli powder**. Continue cooking for 3 or 4 minutes, then add this mixture to the lentil mixture.

When it has cooled a little, add **3 chopped spring onions (scallions)** and **15g (½ cup) yarrow leaves**, stripped off the long stems. This enables them to keep their bright green color. Knead well by hand for about 10 minutes to make a smooth paste. Add **salt** and **pepper** to taste.

With wet hands, shape small balls of the mixture into elongated lozenge shapes, and place on a serving plate with **lettuce leaves** and **wedges of lemon** to squeeze over them. Makes about 12.

Alternative: To make them gluten-free, use cooked quinoa in place of the bulghur.

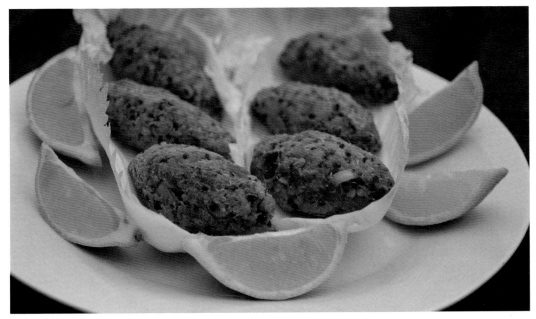

References

Expanded author/date references from the text, plus some of the other works we found useful and inspiring; square brackets indicate other editions and underlining is used for websites

All Year Round Magazine (1859–95), 1876

Allen, David E. & Gabrielle Hatfield (2004). *Medicinal Plants in Folk Tradition: An Ethnobotany of Britain & Ireland.* Portland, OR: Timber Press

American Botanist, The (1901–), 1903

Anon. (c1440). *Two Fifteenth Century Cookery Books.* ed. Thomas Austin. London: Early English Text Society [1888]

Baïracli Levy, Juliette de (1974). *Illustrated Herbal Handbook for Everyone.* London: Faber & Faber

Barker, Julian (2001). *The Medicinal Flora of Britain and Northwest Europe: A Field Guide.* West Wickham: Winter Press

Barstow, Stephen (2014). *Around the World in Eighty Plants.* East Meon: Permanent Publications

Bate, Jonathan (2004). *John Clare: A Biography.* London: Picador [2003]

Baudar, Pascal (2016). *The New Wildcrafted Cuisine: Exploring the Exotic Gastronomy of Local Terroir.* White River Junction, VT: Chelsea Green Publishing

Blair, Katrina (2014). *The Wild Wisdom of Weeds: 13 Essential Plants for Human Survival.* White River Junction, VT: Chelsea Green Publishing

Blamey, Marjorie, Richard Fitter & Alastair Fitter (2003). *Wild Flowers of Britain & Ireland.* London: A&C Black [2013]

Boerhaave, Herman (1741). *Elementa Chemiae*, trans. Peter Shaw. London: T. & T. Longman

Bridges, Robert (1912). *Poetical Works.* London: Oxford University Press

Brill, 'Wildman' Steve (2002). *The Wild Vegan Cookbook: A Forager's Culinary Guide.* Boston, MA: The Harvard Common Press

—— & Evelyn Dean (1994). *Identifying and Harvesting Edible and Medicinal Plants in Wild (and Not So Wild) Places.* New York: A HarperResource Book [2002]

Brinckmann, Josef et al. (2020). Quality Standards for Botannicals. *HerbalGram* 126 (May–June): 50–65

British Herbal Medical Association (1996). *British Herbal Pharmacopoeia.* Exeter: BHMA

Brook, Richard (1800). *A New Family Herbal.* London: W.M. Clark

Bruton-Seal, Julie & Carol Tracy (1988). *Vegetarian Masterpieces* [Charlotte, NC: privately published]

Bryant, Charles (1783). *Flora Diaetetica: Or, History of Esculent Plants, Both Domestic and Foreign.* London: B.H. White

CABI Invasive Species Compendium, www.cabi.org

Carluccio, Antonio (2001). *Antonio Carluccio Goes Wild.* London: Headline Book Publishing

Christopher, John R. (1996). *School of Natural Healing.* Springville, UT: Christopher Publications, Inc. [1976]

Cleghorn, George (1751). *Observations on the Epidemical Diseases in Minorca from the Year 1744 to 1749.* London: T. Cadell

Cocker, Mark (2014). *Claxton: Field Notes from a Small Planet.* London: Jonathan Cape

Coles, William (1656). *The Art of Simpling: An Introduction to the Knowledge and Gathering of Plants.* London: J.G. for Nath. Brook

Commission E (1994). *Yarrow.* American Botanical Council [2000], cms.herbalgram.org

Culpeper, Nicholas (1652). *The English Physitian: Or, an Astrologo-Physical Discourse of the Vulgar Herbs of This Nation.* London: Peter Cole

—— (1653). *Pharmacopoeia Londinensis: Or The London Dispensatory.* London: Peter Cole [first English translation; original in Latin, 1618]

Cummins, Cathal et al. (2018). A Separated Vortex Ring Underlies the Flight of the Dandelion. *Nature* 562: 414–418

Darrell, Nikki (2020). *Conversations with Plants: The Path Back to Nature.* London: Aeon Books [2014]

David, Elizabeth (2013). *On Vegetables*, compiled by Jill Norman. London: Quadrille Publishing

Davidson, Alan (2014). *The Oxford Companion to Food.* 3rd edn, ed. Tom Jaine. Oxford: Oxford University Press [1999]

Domestic Encyclopaedia, The, Or a Dictionary of Facts (1802), 4 vols, ed. A.F.M. Willich. London: Murray & Highley, commons.wikimedia.org

Du Cann, Charlotte (2012). *52 Flowers that Shook My World: A Radical Return to Earth.* Isle of Lewis: Two Ravens Press

Evans, Paul (2019). *Guardian*, Country Diary, 6 June

Evelyn, John (1664). *Sylva, Or A Discourse of Forest-Trees.* London: John Martyn for the Royal Society

—— (1699). *Acetaria: A Discourse of Sallets.* London: B. Tooke

Feehan, John (2009). *The Wildflowers of County Offaly.* Tullamore, Co. Offaly: Offaly County Council

Fern, Ken (2000). *Plants for a Future: Edible & Useful Plants for a Healthier World.* East Meon: Permanent Publications

Fernie, W.T. (1897). *Herbal Simples: Approved for Modern Uses of Cure.* London: Butterworth-Heinemann, wellcomecollection.org

Garrett, J.T. & Michael Garrett (1996). *Medicine of the Cherokee: The Way of Right Relationship.* Rochester, VT: Bear & Company, Inc.

Gerard, John (1597). *The Herball, Or Generall Historie of Plantes.* London: John Norton

—— (1633). *The Herball, Or Generall Historie of Plantes*, ed. Thomas Johnson. London: Adam Islip for Joice Norton & Richard Whitakers

Gibbons, Euell (1962). *Stalking the Wild Asparagus.* Guilford, CT: Alan C. Hood & Company, Inc.

—— (1966). *Stalking the Healthful Herbs.* New York: David McKay Company

Gillam, Fred, thewildsideoflife.co.uk

Gleeson, Erin (2014). *The Forest Feast: Simple Vegetarian Recipes from My Cabin in the Woods.* New York: Abrams

Godwin, H. (1956). *The History of the British Flora: A Factual Basis for Phytogeography.* Cambridge: Cambridge University Press [1984]

Goodman, Adrian M. (2004). Mechanical Adaptations of Cleavers (*Galium aparine*). *Ann. Bot.* 95(3): 475–480. doi: 10.1093/aob/mci038

Gray, Beverley (2011). *The Boreal Herbal: Wild Food and Medicine Plants of the North.* White Horse, Yukon: Aroma Borealis Press

Green Deane (n.d.) Eat the Weeds archive, eattheweeds.com

Grete Herball, The (1526). London: Peter Treveris

Grieve, Mrs M. (1931) *A Modern Herbal.* London: Jonathan Cape [2015], botanical.com

Grigson, Geoffrey (1958). *The Englishman's Flora.* London: Phoenix House [1996]

Hardy, Karen & Lucy Kubiak-Martens, eds (2016). *Wild Harvest: Plants in the Hominin and Pre-Agrarian Human Worlds.* Oxford: Oxbow Books

Harford, Robin (2015). *The Eatweeds Cookbook.* Exeter: Eatweeds, eatweeds.co.uk

Harrap, Simon (2013). *Harrap's Wild Flowers: A Field Guide to the Wild Flowers of Britain & Ireland.* London: Bloomsbury [2018]

Hatfield, Gabrielle (2007). *Hatfield's Herbal: The Secret History of British Plants.* London: Allen Lane

Hawthorne, Nathaniel (1869). *Passages from the American Notebooks.* Boston, MA: Houghton, Mifflin

Hicks, Damien et al. (2016) Food for Pollinators: Quantifying the Nectar and Pollen Resources of Urban Flower Meadows. *PLoS ONE* 11(6): e0158117

Holmes, Peter (1989). *The Energetics of Western Herbs: A Materia Medica Integrating Western and Oriental Herbal Medicine Traditions,* 2 vols. Berkeley, CA: NatTrop [2020]

Hooke, Robert (1665). *Micrographia, or Some Physiological Descriptions of Minute Bodies Made by Magnifying Glasses.* London: Jo. Martyn & Ja. Allestry, Printers to the Royal Society

Hope, Chris (2015). Thistles: A High-Nutrient Weed. *Permaculture* magazine, www.permaculture.co.uk

Hughes, Nathaniel & Fiona Owen (2016). *Weeds in the Heart: A Five Valleys Herbal.* Stroud: Quintessence Press [2018]

Irving, Miles (2009). *The Forager Handbook: A Guide to the Edible Plants of Britain.* London: Ebury Press

Josselyn, John (1672). *New England's Rarities, discovered in Birds, Beasts, Fishes, Serpents, and Plants of that Country.* London: G. Widowes, biodiversitylibrary.org

Jumbalaya, Johnny (2003). *The Essential Hedgerow and Wayside Cookbook.* No place, publisher

Kallas, John (2003). Making Dandelions Palatable. *Backwoods Home* magazine 82, July/August. backwoodshome.com

Kapoor, Sybil (2003). *Taste: A New Way to Cook.* London: Mitchell Beazley

Kew Plant List, theplantlist.org

Lawson, William (1618). *A New Orchard and Garden, with The Country Housewifes Garden,* ed. Malcolm Thick. Totnes: Prospect Books [2003]

Lewis-Stempel, John (2009). *The Wild Life: A Year of Living on Wild Food.* London: Doubleday

Luard, Elisabeth (2007). *European Peasant Cookery.* London: Grub Street [1986]

Lupton, Thomas (1579). *A Thousand Notable Things, of Sundry Sortes.* London: Iohn Charlewood

Lyte, Henry (1578). *A nieuwe Herball, Or, Historie of Plants.* London: Ninian Newton

Mabberley, David J. (2008). *Mabberley's Plant-Book: A Portable Dictionary of Plants, Their Classification and Uses,* 3rd edn. Cambridge: Cambridge University Press [1987]

Mabey, Richard (2010). *Weeds: How Vagabond Plants Gatecrashed Civilisation and Changed the Way We Think About Nature.* London: Profile Books [2012]

Mears, Ray & Gordon Hillman (2007). *Wild Food.* London: Hodder & Stoughton

Mességué, Maurice (1979). *Health Secrets of Plants and Herbs.* London: Collins

Michael, Pamela (1980). *All Good Things Around Us.* London: Ernest Benn [rev. as *Edible Plants & Herbs,* 2015]

Milliken, William & Sam Bridgewater (2013). *Flora Celtica: Plants and People in Scotland.* Edinburgh: Birlinn [2004]

Moore, Michael (1979) *Medicinal Plants of the Mountain West.* Santa Fe, NM: Museum of New Mexico Press

Morency, Pierre (1992). *The Eye is an Eagle: Nature Stories from the New World,* trans. Linda Gaboriau. Toronto: Exile Editions [1989]

Morss, Alex (2020). 'Not Just Weeds': How Rebel Botanists Are Using Graffiti to Name Forgotten Flora. *Guardian,* 1 May

Mother Earth News (1970–), 2011, motherearthnews.com

NAEB (Native American Ethnobotany database), naeb.brit.org

Nearing, Helen (1980). *Simple Food for the Good Life.* Walpole, NH: Stillpoint Publishing

Ó Céirín, Cyril & Kit (1978). *Wild and Free: Cooking from Nature.* Dublin: The O'Brien Press

OED (Oxford English Dictionary) online, oed.com

Packham, Chris (2021). How to Get in Touch with Nature. *The Times,* Weekend, p5, 27 February

Palaiseul, Jean (1973). *Grandmother's Secrets: Her Green Guide to Health from Plants,* trans. Pamela Swinglehurst. Harmondsworth: Penguin Books [1976]

Parkinson, John (1629). *Paradisi in Sole: Paradisus Terrestris, Or, A Garden of Pleasant Flowers.* London: Humfrey Lownes & Robert Young [1976]

—— (1640). *Theatrum Botanicum: The Theater of Plants, Or, An Herball of Large Extent.* London: Tho. Cotes

Pechey, John (1707). *The Compleat Herbal of Physical Plants,* 2nd edn. London: R. & J. Bonwicke [1694]

Phillips, Roger (1983) *Wild Food: A Unique Photographic Guide to Finding, Cooking and Eating Wild Plants, Mushrooms and Seaweed.* London: Pan Books [2014]

—— (1986). *The Photographic Guide to Identify Garden and Field Weeds.* London: Elm Tree Books

Pierpoint Johnson, C. (1862). *The Useful Plants of Great Britain: A Treatise.* London: William Kent & Co.

Pratt, Anne (1866). *Haunts of the Wild Flowers.* London: George Routledge & Sons

Quincy, John (1718). *Pharmacopoeia Officinalis & Extemporanea: Or A Compleat English Dispensatory.* London: Bell

Rees, Gareth E. (2019). *Car Park Life: A Portrait of Britain's Unexplored Urban Wildernesses.* London: Influx Press

Renfrew, Jane M. (1973). *Paleoethnobotany: The Prehistoric Food Plants of the Near East and Europe.* New York: Columbia University Press

Rensten, John (2016). *The Edible City: A Year of Wild Food.* London: Boxtree

RHS (Royal Horticultural Society), rhs.org.uk

Robinson, William (1895). *The Wild Garden.* Portland, OR: Timber Press. Ed. Rick Darke [2009]. Original edn 1870

Roden, Claudia (1968). *A Book of Middle Eastern Food.* Harmondsworth: Penguin Books [1986]

Roth, Sally (2001). *Weeds: Friends or Foe?* London: Carroll & Brown Publishers

Salisbury, Sir Edward (1961). *Weeds & Aliens.* The New Naturalist series 43. London: Collins

Salmon, William (1710). *Botanologia: The English Herbal*, vol. 1. London: H. Rhodes & I. Taylor

Saul, Hayley et al. (2013). Phytoliths in Pottery Reveal the Use of Spice in European Prehistoric Cuisine. *PLoS ONE* 8(8): e70583

Scott, Timothy Lee (2010). *Invasive Plant Medicine: The Ecological Benefits and Healing Abilities of Invasives.* Rochester, VT: Healing Arts Press

Seal, Matthew (2018). Eat Your Weeds! *Herbs* magazine, March, 43.1: 12–13

Sheldrake, Rupert (2020). *Entangled Life: How Fungi Make Our Worlds, Change Our Minds and Shape Our Futures.* London: The Bodley Head

Sherzai, Dean & Ayesha Sherzai (2021). *The 30-day Alzheimer's Solution: The Definitive Food and Lifestyle Guide to Preventing Cognitive Decline.* San Francisco: HarperOne

Shipley, Gerhard P. & Kelly Kindscher (2016). Evidence for the Paleoethnobotany of the Neanderthal: A Review of the Literature. *Scientifica*, article ID 8927654

Sich, Julia, juliasedibleweeds.com

Silverman, Maida (1997). *A City Herbal: Lore, Legend & Uses of Common Weeds.* Woodstock, NY: Ash Tree Publishing [1977]

Stace, Clive (2010). *New Flora of the British Isles*, 3rd edn. Cambridge: Cambridge University Press [1991]

Swift, Jonathan (1710). *Journal to Stella*, ed. George A. Aitken. London: Methuen & Co. [1901], 30 Sept. 1710

Taylor, Rev. Richard (1848). *A Leaf from the Natural History of New Zealand.* Auckland: J. Williamson, natlib.govt.nz

Thompson, Ken (2009). *The Book of Weeds: How to Deal with Plants that Behave Badly.* London: Dorling Kindersley

Thomson, Barbara & Ian Shaw (2002). A Comparison of Risk and Protective Factors for Colorectal Cancer in the Diet of New Zealand Maori and Non-Maori. *Asian Pac. J Cancer Prev.* 3(4): 319–324, PMID 1276290

Thoreau, Henry D. (1865). *Cape Cod.* Boston: Ticknor & Fields

Tobyn, Graeme, Alison Denham and Margaret Whitelegg (2011). *The Western Herbal Tradition: 2000 Years of Medicinal Plant Knowledge.* Edinburgh: Churchill Livingstone [2016]

Tree, Isabella (2018). *Wilding: The Return of Nature to a British Farm.* London: Picador

Turner, Nancy J. (2014). *Ancient Pathways, Ancestral Knowledge: Ethnobotany and Ecological Wisdom of Indigenous Peoples of Northwestern North America.* 2 vols. Montreal & Kingston: McGill–Queen's University Press

Turner, William (1562). *A New Herball*, part II. Cologne: Barckman [1995]

Van Wyk, Ben-Erik & Nigel Gericke (2000). *People's Plants: A Guide to Useful Plants of Southern Africa.* Pretoria: Briza Publications

Viney, Michael (2013). Another Life: Sometimes Stickyback is Just the Weed We Need. *Irish Times*, 24 August 2013

Vogel, Alfred (1989). *The Nature Doctor: A Manual of Traditional and Complementary Medicine.* London: Mainstream [1952]

Weed, Susun (1989). *Wise Woman Herbal: Healing Wise.* Woodstock, NY: Ash Tree Publishing

Weise, Vivien (2004). *Cooking Weeds: A Vegetarian Cookery Book.* Totnes: Prospect Books

Wells, Troth (2010). *The Global Vegetarian Kitchen.* Oxford: New Internationalist

Wilde, Monica, monicawildeforager

Wirngo, Fonyuy et al. (2016). The Physiological Effects of Dandelion (*Taraxacum officinale*) in Type 2 Diabetes. *Rev. Diabet. Stud.* 13(2–3): 113–131

Wood, Matthew (2009). *The Earthwise Herbal: A Complete Guide to New World Medicinal Plants.* Berkeley, CA: North Atlantic Books

Wright, John (2010). *Hedgerow.* River Cottage Handbook No. 7. London: Bloomsbury

—— (2016). *A Natural History of the Hedgerow.* London: Profile Books

Wynne Hatfield, Audrey (1964). *Pleasures of Herbs.* London: The Garden Book Club

Zych, Marcin (2007). On Flower Visitors and True Pollinators. *Plant System. & Evol.* 263: 159–179

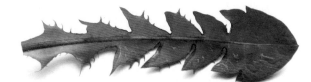

The Forager's Cookbook

Index

Numbers in **bold** indicate main text or recipe references.

The Authors

JULIE BRUTON-SEAL is an herbalist, iridologist and cranio-sacral therapist. A Fellow of the Association of Master Herbalists (FAMH), she is also a photographer, artist, jeweller, graphic designer, cook and gardener. Her parents are the well-known wildlife filmmakers and photographers Des and Jen Bartlett.

MATTHEW SEAL has had a lifelong love of wild flowers, and, like Julie, is a member of the Association of Foragers. By profession an editor and writer in books, magazines and newspapers, he is an Advanced Professional Member of the Chartered Institute of Editing and Proofreading (CIEP).

Julie and Matthew teach courses and workshops in herbal medicine from their base in Norfolk. For more information, see their website: www.hedgerowmedicine.com

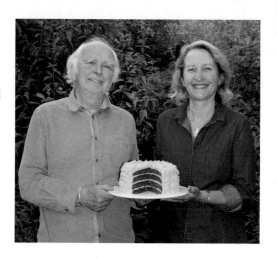

Other books by Julie and Matthew

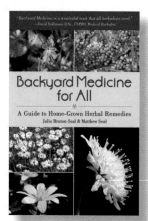

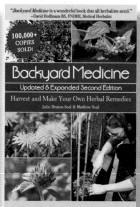

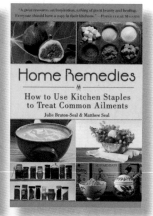

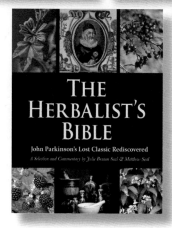

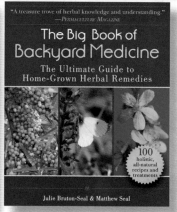

The Forager's Cookbook